Educating
for
Professionalism

Educating
for
Professionalism

Creating a Culture of Humanism in Medical Education

EDITED BY

DELESE WEAR & JANET BICKEL

UNIVERSITY OF IOWA PRESS

IOWA CITY

University of Iowa Press
Iowa City 52242
Copyright © 2000 by the
University of Iowa Press
All rights reserved
Printed in the United States of America

http://www.uiowa.edu/~uipress

The publication of this book was generously supported by the
University of Iowa Foundation.

Printed on acid-free paper

Library of Congress Cataloging-in-Publication Data
Educating for professionalism: creating a culture of humanism in medical education /
Edited by Delese Wear and Janet Bickel.
p.   cm.
Includes bibliographical references and index.
ISBN 0-87745-741-7 (cloth)
1. Medical education—Philosophy.   2. Medical students—Training of.
3. Humanism.   4. Physicians—Attitudes.   5. Medicine—Study and
teaching.   I. Delese Wear.   II. Bickel, Janet W.   III. Title.
R737.W428   2000   610'.71'1—dc21   00-044344

"We are learning when you least expect it."

an anonymous medical student

CONTENTS

JORDAN J. COHEN

Preface

It was Mark Twain who said, "To be good is noble; to teach others to be good is nobler — and less trouble." Of course, the venerable Mr. Twain never ran a medical school. For medical educators, the reverse is true. The challenge of living up to the professional standards we have set for ourselves is certainly great; but the challenge of setting our students on the path to professionalism is even greater.

The Association of American Medical Colleges inaugurated its Initiative on Professionalism in 1998 in response to a growing concern among the public and within the profession that physicians' historical commitment to the tenets of medical professionalism was in danger of withering. Evidence is mounting that the public is increasingly skeptical about the commitment of doctors to place their patients' interests above their own. This alarming trend raises serious questions about the future of the medical profession and has served to stimulate not only the AAMC but many other professional organizations and individual leaders of medicine to redouble their efforts to preserve this critical aspect of our heritage.

The AAMC has launched a multifaceted professionalism initiative which includes a yearlong effort to collect information on precisely how medical schools are going about the teaching of professionalism. Our hope is that this information will be used to develop effective curricular models for helping educators inculcate the values and behaviors composing medical professionalism. Additional assistance is to be found in the journal articles and conference proceedings that have appeared in unprecedented numbers over the past three to four years.

So . . . how are we doing? While reflecting on how we might begin to measure the success of our efforts, I took a look at this important new book. Frederic Hafferty's chapter entitled "In Search of a Lost Cord: Professionalism and Medical Education's Hidden Curriculum" brought me up short with a keen reminder that our success in stressing the importance of lofty values often can be measured using mundane, even commercial tools. He notes the increased level of rhetorical attention that medical educators have devoted to professionalism of late, but then asks us to consider whether or not this heightened emphasis on professionalism is being felt "on the street," so to speak. In other words: what does Stanley Kaplan say?

You know Stanley Kaplan. You know the Princeton Review. These are two of the many outfits that make their living preparing would-be medical students for the MCAT and for the whole medical school admissions process. Their livelihood depends on knowing what qualities medical schools are looking for in a student, and in coaching students how to demonstrate those qualities to admissions committees. As Fred Hafferty points out, if it were true that medical schools were seeking more than academic superstars, and were seriously looking for individuals with the character traits of a caring physician, Stanley Kaplan and his ilk would be the first to jump on the bandwagon. And, at least so far, they haven't. Clearly, we have a lot more work to do.

Fortunately, here is a book that can help a great deal. Delese Wear and Janet Bickel have assembled some of the most accomplished students of the subject to elucidate the many facets of teaching, valuing, and maintaining medical professionalism in the midst of the myriad challenges facing medicine in the early twenty-first century. In addition, they have focused appropriately on *community service* — a critical and expanding aspect of the profession's covenant with the public.

Moreover, this helpful volume could not be coming at a time of greater need. Medical schools and teaching hospitals are being called upon as never before to divert attention away from their core academic purposes in order to meet external challenges to their very survival as educational institutions. As I write this, medical schools and teaching hospitals are engaged in a pitched battle to protect their financial solvency in the face of a fiercely competitive private marketplace and of steep reductions in public funding through Medicare, as mandated by the Balanced Budget Act of 1997.

Continued fiscal stringency, which appears inevitable, adds both urgency and difficulty to maintaining both our professionalism and our community service missions, rendering this volume all the more timely. I hope that the thoughtful reflections and real-world observations provided by the contributors to this book will add needed energy to our pursuit of these critical missions of academic medicine.

DELESE WEAR

Introduction

Why the concern about professionalism in medicine? Throughout the academic medicine community there are calls for attending more vigorously to the professional development of medical students. According to Fred Hafferty, *Academic Medicine* — clearly the premier U.S. journal in medical education — published twenty-five articles focusing on issues of medical professionalism in the three-year period between 1996 and 1998. Even clinical journals such as the *Journal of the American Medical Association*, the *New England Journal of Medicine*, and the *Annals of Internal Medicine* have recently published articles on professional development. What sparked this resurgent attention among medical educators, this sense of urgency about physicians' attitudes and values? What are doctors' obligations to their patients? What are their obligations to the communities where their patients live and work? And what can we do as medical educators to promote and nurture the professional growth of doctors who attend to the needs of individual patients *and* to the larger health needs of communities?

We identified several key areas to explore in this volume. First, we asked contributors to amplify the concept of professional development, a request that yielded surprising coherence. While their orientations toward and experiences with professional development are varied, their definitions are quite similar. Most authors refer to the American Board of Internal Medicine's Project Professionalism and the Association of American Medical Colleges' Medical Schools Objectives Project. The former highlights the values of altruism, accountability, excellence, duty, service, honor, integrity and respect for others, and the evaluation of these qualities. The latter addresses the question "What skills, what attitudes, and what values should every medical student be expected to demonstrate before receiving the M.D. degree?" with learning objectives that each medical school must address in its curriculum. If not citing directly from those sources, other contributors use very similar descriptions of the attributes of professional development.

As Renée Fox observes about past efforts to promote professionalism in medical education, these attempts "contain virtually the same rediscovered principles and qualities of good physicianhood and medical care, the same concern over the degree to which these conceptions are being honored . . . the same explanatory diagnoses of what accounts for [any] deficiencies, along with renewed dedication to remedying them" (1990, p. 201). Thus, we challenged contributors to this volume to address the various sources of and obstacles to professional development more critically. Their responses examine institutional policies (e.g., how and by whom are decisions made?), faculty behaviors (e.g., are they evaluated on their mentoring skills?), curriculum organization (e.g., are there service-learning opportunities?), evaluation practices (e.g., do they further self-reflection?), and the increasing influence of managed care (how are pressures to economize affecting medical education?). Several recurring themes emerged in response to these questions, particularly concerning the influence of the hidden and informal curriculum on students' professional development.

The second key area we asked contributors to explore concerned specific programs and practices implemented in medical education to enhance professionalism. Several contributors describe curricular and other responses to both faculty- and student-identified problems such as cynicism and competitiveness. These responses take the form of programs with a limited life to address specific issues particular to one locale; other responses address professionalism more globally and are systematically threaded throughout the curriculum. Implicit in these accounts is their belief that professional development cannot grow in an environment where it is evaluated but not systematically nurtured.

Much less well charted territory is the relationship between professional development and the health needs of communities. How do the values of altruism and service move beyond the context of medical school ethics courses, student-led task forces, or mentoring programs to the health needs of the public? Do physicians have a responsibility to become health activists in the communities where their patients live and work? In the preface to this book, the AAMC's Jordan Cohen says they do, calling community service "a critical and expanding aspect of the profession's covenant with the public." Students often recognize this covenant and find something vital missing in their medical education: "What they feel is being left out," contributor Edward Eckenfels writes here, "is an affirmation of the core values that motivated them to become physicians in the first place, namely, the moral consciousness, the social responsibility, the idealism that they believe are the foundation of the medical profession." Thus we include four chapters that focus on community-based experiences as an important (and often missing) link in professional development efforts. These chapters address the following questions: What skills, attitudes, and values do medical students acquire in these sites? How are such programs developed, organized, implemented, and maintained? Should all students be required to participate in such programs, or should they be voluntary? What effect do learning experiences in urban classrooms, free clinics, geriatric centers, or HIV support groups have on the professional development of medical students?

To address the intersections of the above queries, we assembled a diverse group of highly respected medical educators, many of whom have decades of experience in these arenas. Paralleling the two key areas detailed above — one critical and theoretical, the other more practice-based — the book is organized into two sections. The first, Understanding the Experience of Medical Education, provides several theoretical considerations that inform the meanings of professionalism. The second, Shaping the Experience of Medical Education, describes specific programs developed by medical educators to enhance the professional development of trainees. The organization of this book, then, reflects multiple vantage points from which professional development is conceived by administrators, faculty, and students as they grapple with its complexities in medical school, clinical, and community contexts.

Part 1, Understanding the Experience of Medical Education, includes four chapters that examine the often conflicting ethical, social, emotional, and intellectual messages medical institutions send to students about what it means to be a doctor. These messages, embedded in admissions policies, the formal, informal, and hidden curricula, grading/evaluation policies, and the clinical training environment, profoundly influence the professional development of medical students and, later, residents. Stanley Joel Reiser's chapter, "The Moral Order of the Medical School," inspects institutional practices, including interactions of all kinds between faculty, staff, and students; institutional policies, rituals, and traditions; and the physical environment itself. The medium is the professional development message, he maintains, and suggests a variety of ways that administrators and faculty can create a more humane environment, such as through institutional grand rounds, where they themselves enact what they expect of students. Through the eyes of a medical student from her admission through graduation, Jack Coulehan and Peter Williams describe how medical education can erode students' idealism and social commitments in their chapter, "Professional Ethics and Social Activism: Where Have We Been? Where Are We Going?" This erosion occurs as a result of several socializing phenomena in medical education, none of which are found in the formal curriculum but which are learned as if they were. These include the development of detachment, a sense of entitlement, and a nonreflective professional practice. One of their hopeful but cautionary remedies is curricular, as they describe their fifty-six-hour interdisciplinary course, "Medicine in Contemporary Society," as a place where professional development can be fostered in both students *and* faculty.

In his chapter, "In Search of a Lost Cord: Professionalism and Medical Education's Hidden Curriculum," Fred Hafferty analyzes our professional development discourse, noting that professionalism has been variously called forth as a historical phenomenon, as a curriculum, as a social label, as a tool for accreditation, and, most recently, as a focus of managed care. Like the other authors in this section, Hafferty strongly believes that medical educators and students need to understand the profound influences of the hidden curriculum — from mission statements to admissions procedures to clinical training rituals. Hafferty concludes that we should work against negative socializing influences by (re)conceiving medicine as a service-oriented occupation. In another chapter of this section, "Professional Role in Health Care Institutions: Toward an Ethics of Authenticity," Richard Martinez also looks critically at institutional environments as they contribute to the diffusion of individual responsibility. He argues that when "professional role" is tied to institutional priorities and goals, students (and clearly all physicians) are discouraged from authentic moral expression when conflict arises between institutions and individuals, stunting professional development. He calls for an "ethics of authenticity" as a critical component of professional development, whereby medical educators support students who identify and question troublesome practices and goals in medical education and in the larger medical community. A common thread of this section is the tenet that professional development efforts will remain mere Band-Aids unless our academic medical centers (and those who lead them) develop and practice the same skills of critical self-scrutiny they expect of professionally developing students.

Part 2, Shaping the Experience of Medical Education, assumes that proactive experiences in medical education — coursework, mentoring relationships, student-initiated activities, service learning and other community-based experiences — stimulate professional growth. Acknowledging the historically sanctioned traditions in medicine and now corporate influences that inhibit students' development as professionals, the six authors in this section argue that professional growth can be nurtured in many formal and informal ways, focusing on the smaller units of change in medical education.

For instance, the University of Kentucky College of Medicine has incorporated professionalism projects throughout the educational continuum. In their chapter, "Student Advocacy for a Culture of Professionalism," Sheila Woods, Sue Fossen, and Lois Nora describe how the medical school facilitates professional behavior across the four years; the project encompasses admissions, cases used throughout the curriculum, resident and faculty development, and extra-curricular activities. Drawing on her deep appreciation of the challenges students face along the way, Norma Wagoner dissects the many elements of professional development in her chapter, "From Identity Purgatory to Professionalism: Considerations along the Medical Education Continuum." Like Woods, Fossen, and Nora, she suggests a variety of ways educators can promote professionalism in mission statements, milestone ceremonies and events, all-class retreats, service learning, and strategies for students' self-assessment.

While many of us limit debates to what we as faculty members can "do" for/on behalf of students to enhance their professional growth, Mary Anne Johnston reminds us that students themselves bring the purest energies to this goal. In her "Reflections on Experiences with Socially Active Students," she describes student-initiated projects that illustrate an acute desire to keep altruism alive, such as the incorporation of multicultural issues into the curriculum, student-led "ward ethics" seminars during clerkships, student-organized orientation experiences for entering students, and efforts to educate faculty guilty of unprofessional behaviors toward women and minority students.

In a chapter entitled "The Mentor-Mentee Relationship in Medical Education: A New Analysis," Tana Grady-Weliky, Cynthia Kettyle, and Edward Hundert focus exclusively on how mentoring can promote professionalism in medical education. Describing the important difference between role model and mentor, the authors provide a Professional Development Grid that illustrates various configurations of the mentor-mentee relationship, depending on the goals and orientations each member of the dyad brings to the relationship. The challenge of these relationships for the mentor who faces an increasingly heterogeneous medical student body is to remain open and respectful to students with different backgrounds and professional goals in the midst of a largely homogeneous academic medical environment.

Judith Andre, Jake Foglio, and Howard Brody take still another approach to professional development programming efforts, turning to the humanities as a vital influence on students' attitudes and values. In "Moral Growth, Spirituality, and Activism: The Humanities in Medical Education," these authors describe efforts to incorporate the teaching of professional behavior throughout the curriculum, focusing on faculty and staff as well as students. They provide great detail on two courses in particular — ethics and spirituality — which seem to go to the heart of professional development and thus, according to their perspective, moral growth. While the former course relies heavily on reasoning, the latter hinges on sustained self-reflection; both, according to the authors, are components essential to ongoing moral growth.

The four final chapters are grouped together to highlight community-based programs that provide students with firsthand experience in working with the health needs of various populations. In "The Case for Keeping Community Service Voluntary: Narratives from the Rush Community Service Initiatives Program," Edward Eckenfels describes a Rush program that matches students' interests and initiatives with the social and health needs of prescribed segments of the Chicago population. He makes a strong case that such community-based programs must be voluntary if they are to provide the real conditions for altruism, duty, and authentic professional development. For some, the effect of these experiences is a reinforcement of what they already believe; for others it is an awakening. Donald Wasylenki, Niall Byrne, and Barbara McRobb describe a *required* half-day community experience spanning the first two years of medical school in their chapter, "Community-Oriented Medical Education: The Toronto Experience." Activities in which students participate include accompanying home health care professionals, working with urban schools and community agencies in health promotion, and studying the interaction of a health problem and a social issue in an agency placement. Their chapter provides extensive detail about organizing and maintaining community learning experiences for large groups of undergraduate students. Similarly, Lucy Tuton, Claudia Siegel, and Timothy Campbell (on behalf of the Bridging the Gaps Network) describe an intensive health-related community service experience in partnership with community organizations administered by representatives from seven of Pennsylvania's eight academic health centers. Their chapter, "Bridging the Gaps: Philadelphia Community Health Internship Program," focuses less on logistics and organization and more on how the program fosters values of collaboration, compassion, communication, tolerance, and accountability. These authors believe, like others in this section, that the best way to impart a conception of the health care professional as a partner with the community he or she serves is *experientially* in locations outside of academic centers.

Another chapter, "Experiencing Community Medicine during Residency: The La Mesa Housecleaning Cooperative," is the story of two family practice residents and their efforts to help form a cooperative composed of Mexican immigrant women from a low-income neighborhood in Albuquerque, New Mexico. Emphasizing health as social, physical, economic, emotional, and spiritual well-being, and not just absence of disease, Fred Miller, Bill Melton, and Howard Waitzkin provide a richly detailed case study in community-oriented health care with significant implications for the values and attitudes espoused in the discourses of professional development.

We have not covered the waterfront here. Many longstanding academic medical centers, their affiliated community health programs, and other relevant work are not detailed. But the authors found here offer a timely, reflective analysis of the work and opportunities facing medical education if medicine is to continue to be trusted by the public. Their chapters remind us time and again that the place to begin is at home, not by medical educators focusing exclusively on the individual medical trainee, but by each academic medical center critically scrutinizing its own environment and the expectations, practices, and behaviors therein that influence the professional development of its students. In an afterword, Janet Bickel offers a summary of the challenges medical educators face in implementing the ideas found here.

Educating
for
Professionalism

PART ONE

Understanding the Experience of Medical Education

STANLEY JOEL REISER

The Moral Order of the Medical School

The moral order of the medical school is created by the interactions among the members of its community, and by the policies and pronouncements it undertakes in the course of institutional governance. The ethical influence of these activities on the people who learn and work in the institution is as profound as that of courses and the other kinds of formal ethical discourse it sponsors. This chapter examines the moral influence of institutional relationships and policies on the life of the medical school and the professional development of its students. In medical education, the medium is indeed the message.

Interactions between Students and Personnel

When teachers present the most pertinent aspects of their field to students and strive to secure the personal involvement of students in the tasks of learning, they fulfill critical requirements of their profession. But what teachers themselves *do* with their knowledge and lives is educationally and morally significant. Do they serve patients without the means to pay for health care through work in community clinics? Do they help the public understand the reach and limits of their fields through popular articles, editorials, or talks? Do they express disagreements with colleagues respectfully? Do they treat staff and professional colleagues beneath and above them in the school's hierarchy with equal dignity? Do they balance their commitments to professional duties and family responsibilities well?

"The Physician," an essay focused on ethics in the Hippocratic writings, depicts the educational importance of the doctor's character and actions. It begins: "The dignity of a physician requires that he should look healthy . . . for the common crowd consider those who are not of this excellent bodily condition to be unable to take care of others. . . . [He should have] a great regularity of life, since thereby his reputation will be greatly enhanced; he must be a gentleman in character, and being thus he must be grave and kind to all" (Hippocrates, 1923b, p. 311). These admonitions do not address patient care itself, but they are highly significant for it, because they predict what kind of care a doctor will give. Who doctors are outside of the medical relationship anticipates who they are likely to be within it. By analogy, what professors do with their knowledge beyond the classroom influences the learning that takes place in it. Students learn to trust their professors from seeing them not just hone, but live, their arguments.

Teachers also influence students by caring about and respecting them. All teaching involves the simultaneous transmission of two lessons: one is a lesson about theory or technique — why nature or artifact is what it is, or how to do something; the second is a lesson about ethics — the teacher's response to the student's efforts to learn and grow. The first lesson teaches students about intellectual constructs and technological reach and limits; the second instructs them about the exercise of power and authority and the meaning of human dignity. Too often teachers focus on the first lesson, either unaware of or unsympathetic to the second. But diminishing the significance of concern and respect in human relationships may be by far the most powerful lesson that teachers leave behind.

The clinic is a particular generator of problems associated with unintended messages. The time demands on clinical teachers, usually residents, often do not allow for much more than just showing students "how to do it." The difficulty for students of using a given technique on frightened, vulnerable, and sometimes inarticulate patients can be lost or ignored by instructors, along with the effect of insensitive criticism of students' efforts should they fail to apply it adequately. All lessons faculty give students affect multiple aspects of their lives, from their immediate development to their future relationships with colleagues and patients.

An exchange of obligations between student and teacher is at the heart of the Hippocratic oath, which creates the concept of profession in Western medicine (Hippocrates, 1923a, pp. 299–301). After the introductory sentence of the oath, which focuses on the solemnity of the act of taking it and the significance of the obligations assumed by those who swear to it, comes a section on the student-teacher relationship. Students are asked to share income with teachers if they are needy, to educate without fee the sons of teachers who wish to learn medicine, and to hold teachers as equal to parents! Such extraordinary commitments emphasize ethical reciprocity as central to the association of students and teachers. The weighty return expected of a student implies a weighty commitment by the teacher in the initial learning process, and a continuing relationship once this stage is over. The student and teacher develop a lifelong bond of care and concern.

·   *Stanley Joel Reiser*

Further, the student-teacher relationship prefigures the student-patient relationship. Students first learn about the use of authority in medicine from the faculty — how those with power and knowledge treat those who lack it. Albert Schweitzer is credited with saying, "Example is not the main thing in influencing others, it is the only thing" (Maudsley, 1999, p. 144). Thus medical educators must help students understand the complexities of relationships with their teachers, recognize that they should not treat students as passive vehicles into whom knowledge is poured, and learn that the teaching relationship carries lessons which influence the human as well as the technical side of the professionals their students become.

How can students help create the feelings and duties of reciprocity found in the oath and thus elevate and bring harmony into their learning relationships? Students must have a commitment to know the subjects they study — not only acquiring basic facts but also appreciating possibilities and shortcomings. Here, students have an advantage over their teachers. Faculty, immersed for years in the normative views of their discipline and writing articles to extend this knowledge, are usually less and less able or willing to see the flaws and inconsistencies potentially visible to new eyes. If faculty are open to it, and students are inclined to question the assumptions of a field, this kind of engagement can create an excitement and mutuality in the learning relationship.

Students should also recognize the ethical issues confronting them in their daily learning. For example, students coming to the bedside of a patient to develop skills in taking a history, doing a physical exam, or drawing blood should acknowledge their limits to patients and follow the "do no harm" ethic. Students must ask patients for permission to learn on them, and patients must give their consent. When students feel they need the help of their teachers in the face of a possible harm to a patient, they should not be afraid to ask for it. Students should be supported when they make the hard choice of seeking assistance. Since most students are concerned about appearing unprepared and indecisive, or challenging the norm of self-reliance with such requests, faculty should come to their aid. Faculty should explicitly tell students that they encourage such requests; that they do not wish learning to be purchased at the expense of harm. Nor should they teach students the lesson that silence is appropriate when the possibility of danger to an innocent and vulnerable person exists. It is just as important for students to understand and be guided by such ethical precepts in learning as it will be later in practice. When students minimize or disregard the ethics of learning, they hamper their own progress toward becoming ethical clinicians.

The learning environment of the medical school is shaped not only by its academicians but also by the multitude of other employees, generally referred to as "staff." The staff are the physiological engines of the institution. They open its doors as well as close and guard them; they direct the flow of materials and information to its units; they give help and receive complaints; they provide aid and take tuition; they make appointments, keep records, maintain infrastructure, and repair damage; they organize and oversee the complex fiscal and administrative systems that make the institution run. Students encounter the staff as much as if not more than their professors. What is their place in the educational experience of students?

The staff is the real community of the institution. They tend always to be there, and in the same place. Staff and their spaces are like the residents in neighborhood stores and houses. I once asked a group of about three hundred employees at my school, "What is your job?" They answered lab technician, employee counselor, internal audit, department secretary, security guard, and so forth. I suggested to them that all these were things they *did*, but that their *job* was to create an institutional environment of respect, consideration, and help in a collective effort to educate and develop humane health care professionals. Each staff member had a specific technical task to fulfill to keep the place running, but they all were bound together in a common educative mission. From doing case rounds with staff concerning issues of institutional culture and governance, I can affirm that staff feel themselves elevated in standing and significance when they recognize they have a role in the education of students.

How can the staff be helped to exercise this role? Institutional recognition, encouragement, and validation that learning in medical school has two distinct and coequal dimensions — a technical and an ethical component — are essential. The staff cannot participate directly in the teaching of technical skills but it does participate in the teaching of ethics. In their interactions with students, the staff show by example how to exercise power and authority. Department secretaries as guardians of appointments and access to professors; financial staff in charge of assuring that student monetary obligations are met or providing assistance to meet them; security guards whose keys provide access to facilities — all of them have opportunities to teach students about treating people with respect and dignity; how to show kindness, tolerance, and patience; how to cope with failure; and how to handle success. This cross-section of the real-world community in which the medical student will work and provide care has an enormous potential to educate. Ideally, the medical school should give staff the charge and help to do it, by formally declaring and encouraging the staff in this role, by developing literature and seminars for them on these issues, and by acknowledging in public statements and in salaries particularly meritorious staff-student relationships.

Policies and Pronouncements of the Medical School

The medical school has a moral character independent of, though influenced by, the moral character of those who live in it. The medical school creates its character by the choices and decisions it makes over time as an institution. These actions, which tend to be based on its dominant traditions and values, define the institution to both its members and the public.

A school's history has a major influence on its institutional identity. On the walls of its most significant spaces hang portraits of founders, benefactors, administrators, and professors, and photographs of classes, buildings, and notable events. These displays indicate the relationship of the past to the present. Past accomplishments modulate into school traditions, which establish an identity in the present as elements of the school's reputation. The identity of an institution also derives from the actions of the people presently there. For example, as Norma Wagoner writes in part 2, medical schools all over the country have recently established "white coat" ceremonies, in which first- or second-year students receive this symbol of the medical profession in a ceremony invoking compassion and humility. In addition to such practices, the policies and procedures of medical schools establish or maintain a particular identity.

The collective effect of these events and traditions on those working and learning in the institution is profound. Indeed, they create its master teacher, the institutional ethos. Because its origins are so widespread in place and time, the ethos exerts its influence ubiquitously and invisibly on the policies and actions of the school.

I once was approached by a high administrative officer of a medical school, a physician, to discuss where in the curriculum he might do some teaching, because he really missed it. At the time I too believed in the basic educational dichotomy between administration and faculty, and did my best to help him choose a good class in which to participate. Given that same request from him now, my response would be different. I would suggest that the opportunity to teach is not restricted to the instruction of students in a classroom or clinic. I would point out to the administrator that when he creates and oversees budgets, policies, and educational initiatives, and influences by these actions the communities within and outside of the school, he teaches powerful lessons. I would say that his role as an institutional leader provides an unparalleled visibility and platform from which to instruct the organization's community about matters such as the stewardship of resources, the humane use of authority, the role of values in making judgments, the exercise of patience and courage under duress, how to admit mistakes, how to forgive them, the application of knowledge in taking action, the balance of personal and professional commitments, and so forth.

It is critical that institutional leaders be self-conscious in their roles as teachers and aware of the linkage between policy making and education. It also is important for them to include the institution's constituents in the crafting of policies, as an affirmation of its commitment to open discussion. Institutions show their respect for the dignity and experience of their constituents by giving those affected by choices a voice in helping to shape and decide them. I don't mean by this always seeking to fill auditoriums to decide issues, although this may sometimes be advisable. I mean doing things such as using focus groups of institutional personnel to test ideas; inserting policy questions where appropriate in student forums; using weekly newsletters to alert the community to problems and to ask for suggestions; periodically revising the institutional mission statement in consonance with changing constituent views of school goals; encouraging administrative and departmental units to have periodic meetings about the character of life within them and the school; focusing on hierarchical behavior in the institution to determine how authority is used in academic and staff relationships; asking how the school interacts with its neighborhood and whether this relationship needs change; and so forth.

In constructing its policies, the medical school has an opportunity to fashion its actions on the same foundation that it endeavors to teach in class to its students — the foundation of ethics. The standards that bind physicians together as a profession, that distinguish medicine from business, and that enable individuals when sick to place themselves in a physician's hands constitute the ethics of medicine. If students are urged to use these ethical standards as beacons of right action, shouldn't the institution that educates them do the same?

In illustration of this, let us examine one of the major institutional challenges facing American medical schools — how to survive financially without undermining their educational and service missions. Buffeted by the loss of practice income in the 1990s under the ethos of competition for patients with managed care organizations, and the growing unwillingness of private and governmental payers to factor education time into fee schedules, medical schools have responded with policies under which clinical faculty devote ever increasing amounts of time to reimbursable patient care to make up the revenue shortfall. This in turn has reduced the time they can give to teaching, research, and institutional and community service. Concurrently, many schools have expanded the bureaucracy concerned with practice faster than other aspects of their mission, thereby changing its direction and character.

What ethical consequences flow from the current focus on business and profits? Inevitably, in such an environment, marketplace concerns and values begin to vie with academic and professional ones as the basis for institutional choices. This conflict generates a decidable question: What organizational structure for faculty practice is most compatible with the school's academic obligations and goals? For example, should medical schools become administratively divided into self-sustaining but connected practice, research, and educational domains, where occupants can fully commit themselves to the values and time demands of each domain, but also participate with each other through specified exchanges of expertise and time? Or can a single medical school domain accommodate any longer the diverse interests and ethical values of modern health care?

At the heart of the current crisis is the growing embrace by medical schools of a business ethos reminiscent of pre-Flexnerian times, when the schools viewed themselves as profit centers and integrated education into the business concerns of private practitioners. The reform of medical education in the early twentieth century, guided by Abraham Flexner and innovative ideas from the newly formed Johns Hopkins Medical School (1893), resulted in the creation of an academic and noncommercial focus in medical schools and the development of a limited number of full-time and tenured professorships, whose holders were solely to serve and nurture the infrastructure of learning and research. It is now argued widely that a business focus is needed by modern medical schools to generate financial resources to preserve their educational and scientific activities. Ironically, devoting so much faculty and administration time to achieving success in the practice competition of the marketplace redirects the school's energy and attention away from the very academic programs and objectives this policy was meant to save.

The profound influence of this issue on the work and academic culture of the school requires a broad and open discussion of options. This discussion should consider how alternative choices of action reflect the stewardship responsibilities of the school to preserve not just the institution as a physical entity, but the qualities and values that constitute its core identity as a place to teach and model the attributes of intellectual courage, bedside humaneness, and service to people. To maintain a medical school that has lost its inner content is to maintain its shell, not its essence.

To explore this and other organizational problems in a comprehensive and interactive manner, the case round is an excellent vehicle. Just as practicing physicians test clinical choices and ethical decisions through regularly held case discussions, organizations can do the same. In one approach to this process, institutional problems are converted into cases, which are presented to its constituents. With the help of a moderator, they formulate the key issues raised in the case, which are written down in the order received. The audience discusses these questions and formulates policy issues in need of consideration by the institution. Summaries of these discussions, along with emerging recommendations, are sent to organization leaders (Reiser, 1994).

Medical schools also should consider the development of codes of ethics specifying the values and purposes that will undergird their decisions. The code provides an ethical profile that reflects and selects from the values held by a school's constituents. The medical school needs a formal statement of ethical purpose because its actions influence lives and society in ways that are independent of the individuals who make up the medical community. The divergent values held by these individuals cannot operate effectively to guide institutional actions. Codes differ from institutional mission statements. Codes explicitly focus on ethical standards to guide the institution's daily choices. Mission statements focus on broad, institutional, programmatic goals. These goals, of course, carry ethical messages, and they should be carefully crafted to reflect institutional values.

———

The moral order of the medical school is constructed of relationships — among students, faculty, and staff — which have an ethical content, and of the policies of the institution that enlist its personnel and resources on behalf of particular ends, which in turn make ethical statements. This moral order identifies, as much as any characteristic of the school, what the school is and what it stands for. How well the community of the school creates a moral order will have a profound influence on how well it meets its problems. The inner strength of this community is sustained by a developed and tested capability for mutual trust; by a concern for dignity, consent, and humaneness in institutional relationships; by a commitment to the open discussion of institutional choices; and by a recognition that actions, including the action of silence, reveal moral purpose and create responsibilities. These and other moral values that the community of the medical school may wish to discuss and embrace in its work together are its most basic gifts to its members, and to society. Society will reap the benefits of the school's moral order from the students it educates, the knowledge it generates, and the example it sets for other social institutions about the meaning of serving others.

Stanley Joel Reiser

FREDERIC W. HAFFERTY

In Search of a Lost Cord

Professionalism and Medical Education's Hidden Curriculum

Robert Michels recently wrote that

> it is possible to shape a doctor's behavior so that he or she fits into the desired behavior of a managed care system, but if the doctor does not have it in his soul, his replication of the desired pattern does not work very well. The nurturance of the physician's soul is the function of medical education, and during the chaotic transition between where we are and where we are going, we are putting more capital and effort into redesigning the organization and economic structure of the health care system than into revising the educational system to create the optimal physicians to participate in health care. At present, most medical schools are training doctors who will not be well prepared to practice in the new system. (Michels, 1996)

This statement by Robert Michels is rife with irony. On the one hand, it articulates a fundamental truism for sociologists who study the training of physicians. Socialization is a process by which the self is transformed. Socialization involves the internalization of a new value system, including new ways of thinking, viewing, and talking about things. It truly is about "soul." But Michels also appears to urge medical schools to create better souls for the practice of medicine in managed care settings and to do so at a time when the public has become increasingly concerned about the "motives" and "dangers" of managed care medicine (USA Snapshots, 1999).

The mission statement below and its related list of required coursework contain their own set of ironies. They were selected somewhat capriciously (i.e., the author once worked at the school selected) from the *1998 AAMC Curriculum Guide*, a compendium of the required curricula provided by the 142 allopathic medical schools in the United States ($N = 126$) and Canada ($N = 16$). The mission statement is reproduced verbatim while the course list has been rearranged to make the school's identity more opaque. These two statements of organizational purpose and action are worthy of our attention for several reasons. They function as elemental statements about what it means to be a physician and how individual medical schools should direct their pedagogical efforts. Second, they function as visions of medicine as a profession and the physician as a professional person. Finally, one might reasonably assume that they operate in tandem and that their interdependence is discernible to the casual observer.

_____ School of Medicine provides an educational environment that encourages intellectual diversity and offers stimulation and opportunity for self-motivated students. The curriculum for students in the M.D. program has a twofold purpose: to develop in all students the capacity for leadership in the clinical practice of scientific medicine, and to prepare as many students as possible for careers in research and teaching in the various branches of basic, clinical, and social medicine.

The program of study emphasizes the faculty's belief that medical education should prepare a physician for a lifetime of continued learning. The curricular flexibility of the M.D. program allows students to pursue individual career goals and to develop special interests.

Biochemistry (68 hours)
Biostatistics (24 hours)
Cells and Tissue (75 hours)
Clinical Immunology (18 hours)
Computers in Medical Education (8 hours)
Hematology (30 hours)
Host-Parasite Interaction and Host Defense (27 hours)
Human Anatomy and Embryology (204 hours)
Human Genetics (40 hours)
Infectious Basis of Disease (71 hours)
Introduction to Clinical Problem Solving (121 hours)
The Nervous System (78 hours)
Pathology (152 hours)
Pathophysiology (10 hours)
Pharmacology (89 hours)
Physicians and Patients (30 hours)
    [Includes Nutrition, Cultural Aspects, Sexuality, Prevention]
Physiology (225 hours)
Preparation for Clinical Medicine (132 hours)

Family Medicine (4 weeks)
Gynecology and Obstetrics (4 weeks)
Medicine (8 weeks)
Other Clinical Electives (12 weeks)
Pediatrics (8 weeks)
Psychiatry (4 weeks)
Selective Clerkships (12 weeks)
Surgery (8 weeks)

In the mission statement above, the physician is depicted as a "clinical leader," a researcher, and an academic. "Continued learning" is represented as essential to all these roles. Finally, the ability to pursue "special interests" and "individual career goals" is framed as intrinsic to physicianhood. The list of required coursework, however, does not highlight any of these roles or identities. Leadership, research, and teaching are not formally mentioned. The physician-as-professional also receives no formal mention in either the mission statement or the course list.

These lacunae are significant because they prompt us to ask, Where within the curriculum are we to find pedagogical efforts directed toward what medicine so emphatically proclaims to be its end product, the "caring and competent professional"? If medicine truly harbors that "fundamental specialness" so valued by Relman (1998) and others, where can we go within the training process to see this essence being nurtured? As I will argue in the body of this chapter, becoming a professional takes shape more within medicine's informal and hidden curriculum than within its formally identified teaching modules (Hafferty, 1998; Hafferty & Franks, 1994; Hundert, 1998; Wear, 1997). Furthermore, and perhaps most disconcerting, the norms and value orientations encountered by students during their training are not always the standards medicine ritualistically identifies as defining medical practice.

In the subsequent sections of this chapter, I will explore how the concept of professionalism has been approached within the medical educational literature and how medical schools instruct their trainees, both intentionally and unwittingly, about what it means to be a "medical professional." Within this discussion, I will highlight the medical school as a moral community and training as a process of moral enculturation. I will close with suggestions for how issues of professionalism might be better addressed within medical training, particularly as we move more aggressively into an era of managed care.

For over 150 years, organized medicine has been unrelenting in its quest for professional status. Medicine's efforts in this respect have rested on three assertions. First, medical work is grounded in a unique and esoteric body of scientific knowledge. Second, and because of this knowledge, medical work can be evaluated and regulated only from within — that is, by other physicians. Third, and again based on this claim of an esoteric knowledge base, organized medicine must exercise control over the work of other (and potentially competing) health occupations. In return for this exemption from external review (autonomy) and for the powers associated with occupational dominance, medicine has promised to use its special skills in the service of patients. More specifically, medicine promised to act as a fiduciary, placing the welfare of patients ahead of its own. Medical schools (which would evolve into "medical centers" and then into "academic health centers") were to be the principal site of training (the transmission of knowledge and skills) and socialization (the internalization of important professional attitudes and values) (see Jonas, 1978; Ludmerer, 1985).

Much of the century between 1850 and 1950 stands as testimony to medicine's increasing hegemony. Although there were notable setbacks (e.g., medicine's longstanding attempt to quash chiropractic), it would take the inflationary decade of the 1970s — the twentieth century's longest bear stock market — and the introduction of Medicare and Medicaid in the 1960s, among other social pressures, to signal medicine's diminishing fortunes (Rothman, 1991; Rothstein, 1972; Shryock, 1967; Sigerist, 1935; Starr, 1982; Stevens, 1971). Most recently, the rise of for-profit managed care has raised compelling questions about the future status of medicine as a profession (Hafferty & Light, 1995). In response, organized medicine has waged a vigorous counteroffensive designed to bolster its sagging social legitimacy, its crumbling legal protections, and its deteriorating position as the nation's preeminent profession. We read, for example, that medical schools face a fundamental challenge in helping to restore public trust in medicine *as a profession* (Wallace, 1997; emphasis mine). Camanisch (1988) argues that medicine's current crisis of professionalism is not connected to a loss of knowledge, skills, or overall technical competence, but to its loss of moral standing and authority. During the three-year period of 1996–1998, more than twenty-five articles headlining issues of medical professionalism were published in the Association of American Medical Colleges' journal *Academic Medicine*, most coming in the latter two years.[1,2] Analogous articles appeared in the *New England Journal of Medicine* (Hughes, Barker, & Reynolds, 1994) and the *Journal of the American Medical Association* (Lundberg, 1991; McArthur & Moore, 1997; Ring, 1991; Todd, 1991). The president of the AAMC, Jordan J. Cohen, labeled professionalism intrinsic to the "sanctity of the doctor-patient relationship," and essential to the "very survival" of medicine. Most recently, Cohen identified professionalism as a basic element in the AAMC's latest initiative, the Medical School Objectives Project (see Cohen, 1998a, 1998b, 1998c; AAMC, 1998; The Medical School Objectives Writing Group, 1999).

Despite all of this historical and contemporary attention, a core understanding of what it means to be a professional remains elusive. Although several recent articles have delivered extensive details about core curricula in "professional skills and perspectives" (Curry & Makoul, 1998; Fields, Toffler, Elliot, & Chappelle, 1998; Makoul & Curry, 1998; Makoul, Curry, & Novack, 1998; Steele & Susman, 1998; Wilkes, Usatine, Slavin, & Hoffman, 1998), particulars about *what* is being transmitted — and, one hopes, internalized — remain sketchy. For example, we are told that exemplar courses contain modules in ethics, humanities, and the behavioral sciences, as well as medical economics, population-based medicine, health promotion and disease prevention, physical examination, clinical reasoning, clinical diagnosis, law and medicine, and the latest rage, evidence-based medicine (see Makoul et al., 1998). Similarly, we are informed that these courses are essential in moving medical students "from being experts in applied biosciences to being physicians" (Makoul & Curry, 1998). Additionally, we hear that they foster an understanding of "the roles of physicians in their relationships with patients, the community, and society at large" (Curry & Makoul, 1998), or that they allow students to acquire "an understanding of the larger social and economic problems and trends with which medicine must deal" (Rappleye, 1932). All the above appear to be worthy goals, but they do not constitute definitions of professionalism. Finally, medical students, along with the general public, are told with numbing regularity that the physician-patient relationship is "professional" in nature, that medical education imparts "professional knowledge and skills," and that transmission happens within a particular dynamic ("professional growth"/"professional development").

Within this deluge of claims, the "what" (What makes a relationship "professional"? What does it mean to "act unprofessionally"?) receives far less attention than the "how" (e.g., interdisciplinary coursework, white coat ceremonies, mission statements, graduation oaths). None of the schools formally identified in the January 1998 issue of *Academic Medicine* as having developed "comprehensive coursework in professional skills and perspectives" use any form of the term *professional* in their course title (Oregon Health Sciences University, "Principles of Clinical Medicine"; University of California, Los Angeles, "Doctoring"; Northwestern University, "Patient, Physician and Society"; and University of Nebraska, "The Integrated Clinical Experience").[3] Furthermore, when these schools were asked to present evidence of outcomes, the information provided was at best apologetic and at worst oblique (e.g., details about the form of evaluation [OSCEs, oral and written feedback, or "short-answer or essay tests"] but without specifics relating these measurements to "professionalism"). It appears that medical educators are fast becoming masters of delivering a product no one can define.

———

Possibly underscoring this enigma is the fact that the concept of professionalism has become associated with a daunting array of social actions. Medical education, we are informed, involves "personal growth and professional development," indicating (at the risk of being redundant) that "personal growth" and "professional development" are distinguishable entities. Similarly, medical educators routinely insist that medicine is rife with "ethical and professional dilemmas," implying, once again, that there is a distinction, this time between dilemmas of an "ethical" versus those of a "professional" nature (the same is also true for notions like "unethical and unprofessional conduct").[4] Concurrently, the term "professional" is being used more as an adjective than as a noun. As such, it has come to indicate a certain type of dedication ("professional commitment"), moral stance ("professional values"), social environment ("professional culture"), or approach to work (in a "professional manner"). The label "professional" has been expropriated by other occupational groups to promote an image of expertise and dedication (e.g., "professional landscapers," "professional plumbers") or high quality in work performance ("professional installation," a "professional finish").

———

The enigmatic nature of professionalism is also apparent within the process of medical school accreditation. Although the principal instruction document used by the Liaison Committee on Medical Education (LCME), *The Function and Structure of a Medical School*, contains several references to medicine as a profession (e.g., it calls upon medical schools to instill in its graduates "the values and attitudes consistent with a compassionate professional"; it states that physicians should have a "dedication to service" and that medical schools should educate physicians who will meet the "total medical needs of patients" and gain the "trust and respect of patients, colleagues, and the community"), the princi-

Frederic W. Hafferty

pal data-gathering tool used by the LCME to compile information about individual schools, *The Medical Education Database*, does not require schools to supply information on how they seek to instill (or even evaluate) these values and attitudes.

A recent study by the AAMC of its own accreditation activities (see Kassebaum, Eaglen, & Cutler, 1997) fortifies these observations. In this study, schools judged to have "robust institutional objectives" (meaning schools that had identified "specific domains of knowledge, understanding, skills, and behaviors that students were expected to acquire and be able to exhibit") were awarded this designation because their students had demonstrated basic science and clinical knowledge and skills, including "a broad, comprehensive biopsychosocial approach in the evaluation and care of patients," and "high ethical principles and standards in all aspects of medical practice." However, outside of this reference to high ethical principles and standards (which may or may not stand as synonyms for professionalism — see above) no explicit reference is made to the concept of professionalism, nor to concepts like "caring," "service," or fiduciary obligation, in this rating system. Other studies of the accreditation process (Kassebaum, Cutler, & Eaglen, 1997) stress the importance of measuring knowledge, clinical skills, and "behavior" while terms like "attitudes and values" are conspicuously absent from the assessment equation. Fifteen years ago, the "foremost recommendation" (as identified in Kassebaum et al., 1997) of the GPEP (General Professional Education of the Physician) Report called upon medical education to "emphasize the acquisition and development of skills, values, and attitudes by students at least to the same extent that they do their acquisition of knowledge" (Muller, 1984). In an era when the measurement of outcomes has become a major rallying cry within medical education circles, it appears that medical educators remain fundamentally ambivalent about assessing what supposedly stands as their raison d'être — professionalism. Instead, medical educators prefer to frame professionalism as a skill and/or a behavior devoid of any reference to the "messy" presence of values or attitudes. But even when remaining within the safe harbor of "behavior," medical educators appear to be at a loss as to whether professionalism should be approached as a dichotomous (present/absent) or a continuous level variable and, if the latter, what it means to be "more or less" a professional.

———

Over the past decade, managed care companies have become quite vocal about the failure of medical schools to prepare physicians to practice effectively within organizational systems that focus on care management, interdisciplinary practice, health promotion, and the delivery of services that are evidence-based, outcome-oriented, and cost-effective (Wood, 1998). These companies claim that they are being forced to hire physicians who take upward of two years to acquire the requisite skills, knowledge, and value orientations to work effectively (Shine, 1996). So confronted, managed care companies have begun to suggest that medical schools adopt a rather extensive list of "remedial" coursework covering subject areas such as the organization and financing of health care, resources allocation and risk management, quantitative methods related to the health of populations (e.g., epidemiology, biostatistics, and decision analysis), health services research skills, computer applications and medical informatics, social and behavioral sciences, and medical ethics, among the topics frequently mentioned (see Group Health Association of America, 1994). Again, the notion of professionalism is conspicuously absent.

Organized medicine has not been silent in the face of these criticisms and suggestions. Invoking terms and concepts more often seen in the sociological than the medical literature, medical insiders have denounced the "commodification" of health care by contrasting the "culture of commercialism" versus the "culture of medicine" (McArthur & Moore, 1997; also see Frankford & Konrad, 1998; Lundberg, 1990).[5] Others have contrasted the ideals of profit and competition with those of service, advocacy, and altruism (Langley, 1997; Stone, 1997; Swick, 1998).[6] Medical insiders no less prominent than Arnold Relman (1998) anguish about the conflict between "traditional professional values and the imperatives of the market" and call for "education to defend professional values in the new corporate age."

These antiphons, while heavily infused with rhetoric and ideology, are important to our efforts to understand the nature of professionalism because they contain references missing from articles that detail teaching methods and pedagogy. These cries of outrage and angst contain some rather provocative insights into the nature of professionalism and what it means to act and work in a professional manner. The table below, for instance, summarizes two different lists of "remedial" coursework. The column on the left reflects the findings of a national survey "to define a new core curriculum to prepare physicians for managed care practice" (Meyer, Potter, & Gary, 1997).[7] The second list, offered by Relman (1998), focuses on "professional values." The lists are not organized in a point-counterpoint fashion but represent a simple ordering of attributes as presented in the articles.

Frederic W. Hafferty

A Managed Care Curriculum	A Professional Values Curriculum
1. Health care economics 2. Managed care ethics and medical jurisprudence 3. Information systems 4. Communication skills 5. Decision-analysis skills and biostatistics 6. Technology assessment 7. Managed care essentials (including definitions, concepts, population-based medicine, and preventive medicine) 8. Customer relations 9. Multidisciplinary team building	1. The social and political history of medicine as a profession 2. The economic dimensions of health care 3. The history of health maintenance organizations 4. The political and social underpinnings of the Clinton health care reform efforts 5. The conflicts between the culture of business and the culture of clinical medicine 6. The ethical, legal, and professional challenge of medical industrialization 7. The political and professional options for preserving medical professionalism

These two registers have obvious differences. The managed care list is more technically oriented while the professional values list draws more heavily upon history and sociology. The managed care curriculum does not mention (or even allude to) professionalism. It does, however, introduce readers to a new form of ethics ("managed care ethics"). Relman's curriculum, while highlighting the concept of professionalism, uses the concept more as an adjective ("professional challenge," "professional values") than as a noun. Nonetheless, Relman's embrace of the social sciences does demonstrate how they may serve as important sources of understanding about professionalism, and it is to these frames of reference that we now turn.

Frames of Reference: Sociology, Philosophy, and Ethics

The references to attributes and endeavors such as service, advocacy, and altruism by medical insiders such as Relman (1998) and McArthur and Moore (1997) have their roots in two academic disciplines. The first, academic sociology, has analyzed in great detail the rise (and current fall) of organized medicine as a profession (Hafferty & McKinlay, 1993a; see subsequent citations). The second subject area, covering philosophy and ethics, has focused more on the essential moral nature of the physician-patient relationship (see Flores, 1988; Kultgen, 1988; Moline, 1986; Pellegrino, Veatch, & Langan, 1991). A highly insightful review of these two approaches can be found in Cruess and Cruess's *Academic Medicine* article, "Teaching Medicine as a Profession in the Service of Healing" (1997). Without attempting to summarize this article, and with a brief expansion of the historical points made earlier in this chapter, the following points are noteworthy.

Sociology's initial interest in professionalism and professions emerged in the closing decades of the nineteenth century. This interest corresponded to the rise of an industrialized economy, the emergence of science as the exemplar of rational thought, and the challenge posed by science to traditional belief systems such as religion (Aron, 1967). For example, writing in his second major publication, *Les formes élémentaires de la vie religieuse*, Emile Durkheim saw the rise of a professional class as a necessary response to the growth of industrialization, the rise of an urban underclass, and the increasing differentiation and segmentalization of modern society. For Durkheim, the state had become too remote from the individual while the family had become too narrow a source of influence, having lost its economic function. For these reasons, Durkheim envisioned political order through the creation of intermediary bodies, with professional organizations being the only social groups able to foster the integration of individuals into a collectivity while also protecting the individual from oppression by the state. In what might be considered the ultimate irony, Durkheim interchangeably used the term "corporation" and "profession" while advancing his arguments.

In the ensuing decades, sociology's interest in the professions grew with the discipline. Sociology began to see medicine's rise to professional prominence as being grounded in a variety of social forces. Faced with a host of competitors in the 1880s (e.g., homeopathy, naturalism, and later chiropractic, among others), organized medicine argued that it should be granted legally based privileges and protections so that it could function as the sole source and arbiter of "medical" work. As noted above, this demand had two components: *dominance* over the work of others (usually competitors) and *autonomy*, so that medicine and medicine alone would have control over the terms and conditions of this work, including the selection, training, and licensing of medical practitioners, and most important, the review and evaluation of the work performed by *its* practitioners.

In return for these privileges, powers, and protections, medicine promised *not* to use its dominance and autonomy to further its own ends. Instead, it promised to act in a *fiduciary* manner.

The history of medicine, although rife with accomplishments, is also a history of how medicine has used its monopolistic powers to expand its base of privilege and influence (Rothman, 1991; Starr, 1982). By the 1970s, considerable literature had been amassed documenting medicine's predatory predilections, along with its chronic failure to act in the public's best interests (Barber, 1963; Barzun, 1978; Collins, 1979; Illich, 1976; Larson, 1977; Moore, 1970; Schiedermayer & McCarthy, 1995). As medicine began to lose its bedrock of cultural legitimacy and prestige (Mechanic, 1985), sociologists began to detail a process of deprofessionalization (Haug, 1988), proletarianization (McKinlay & Arches, 1985), and corporatization (Light, 1993). As documented most persuasively by Eliot Freidson (who, incidentally, did not endorse either the proletarianization or deprofessionalization arguments), medicine's lack of external accountability promoted an insidious state of insularity that, in turn, facilitated internally generated myths about medicine's own altruistic motives and actions (Freidson, 1994). In short, the autonomy medicine so coveted created a dialectic. As medicine wandered from its promise to reflect critically on its own actions and motives, it lost the ability to regulate itself in anyone's interests but its own. Most recently, Freidson and others have called for a resurgence of professionalism (as opposed to professional powers) with the goal of reversing medicine's slide from professional grace. In these writings, the characteristics and traits of commitment, a fiduciary relationship, trustworthiness, and discretionary decision making are prominently featured.

Central to this overall literature (see Goode, 1969) is a definition of professionalism as something that resides in the interface between the possession of specialized knowledge and a commitment to use that knowledge for the betterment of others (that is, service). Although medicine successfully sought to transform its earlier promise to act as a fiduciary (to place the welfare of others ahead of one's own welfare) into a promise to act paternalistically (to act in the other's best interests), it was medicine's rejection of help-as-obligation in favor of help-via-philanthropy (aptly characterized by May [1975] as the "conceit of philanthropy") that helped to set the moral tone for what it means to be a professional — at least within the world-view of medicine (see Hafferty & McKinlay, 1993b).

Work within the fields of philosophy and ethics has created its own set of insights into the nature of professionalism and what it means to be a professional. Here the focus has been on the physician-patient relationship, particularly the fiduciary nature of this relationship (Bayles, 1989; Kultgen, 1988; Pellegrino & Thomasma, 1981). More recently, issues of trust have appeared within the literatures of ethics (Flores, 1988; Pellegrino et al., 1991) and sociology (Gray, 1997; Hafferty, 1991; Mechanic & Schlesinger, 1996). Related characteristics include devotion to the public good, virtue (and virtuousness), beneficence, the absence of malfeasance, and the argument that a professional work (or the work of professionals) should be grounded in a "calling" and predicated on personal commitment and a core value set (often operationalized by the profession in a "code of ethics"). Additional terms and concepts include "responsibility" (including the responsibility to be competent and to regulate oneself as a fiduciary), the notion that occupying the status of professional is not a right but a privilege, and the core notion that being a professional entails certain "obligations." Cruess and Cruess (1997), for example, identify eleven obligations covering issues of knowledge and skills (e.g., maintaining competence, ensuring the integrity of the knowledge base, familiarity with codes of professional behavior and national and regional laws and regulations), along with related attitudes, values, and behaviors (e.g., participation in health issues pertaining to social problems, commitment to a fiduciary orientation to medical work).

With these two frames of knowing (sociology and ethics), we now can return to an exploration of how professionalism is handled within the medical literature. While most discussions have taken place within such vaporous distinctions as "science" versus "art" or by invoking emotionally evocative entities such as the alleged "sacred bond" between doctor and patient, there have been attempts to deal with the concept in a more forthright manner. Emanuel (1997), for example, in an attempt to offer "a truer and more helpful" (but ultimately more "medical") definition of professionalism, defines *profession* as "the expert protection of vulnerable people and vulnerable values" with self-regulation "a necessary vehicle for maintaining expert standards." For Emanuel, sociology proposes an alternative — and inferior — definition, with its view of professionalism as the exchange of expertise for self-regulation. In the same issue of *JAMA*, McArthur and Moore (1997) define professional medical care as "the assumption of *responsibility* for the patient's welfare" (emphasis mine) with the "essential image" of the professional being "a practitioner who values the patient's welfare above his or her own and provides services even at a fiscal loss and despite physical discomfort or inconvenience." In their article "Teaching Professionalism: Passing the Torch" (1998), Hensel and Dickey define professionalism as a "public trust" manifested by the presence of "responsible ethical codes" and the elevation of service over proprietary interests. The American Board of Internal Medicine (ABIM) defines professionalism as "aspiring toward altruism, accountability, excellence, duty, service, honor, integrity, and respect for others" (*Project Professionalism*, 1995). On a broader level, McCurdy and colleagues (1997) argue that the relationship of academic medicine and society is a "social contract" and a "social compact," based on trust and covenantal in nature.

In advocating a system of medical education built around professional values, Relman (1998) highlights elements like beneficence, autonomy, and fiduciary responsibility for patients. In 1991, James Ring made professionalism the cornerstone of his presidential address to the American Medical Association ("The Right Road for Medicine: Professionalism and the New American Medical Association"), while defining it as dedication to competence, compassion, and moral accountability along with patient advocacy, "personal sacrifice," and beneficence. The AMA executive vice president, James S. Todd (1991), stresses issues of honesty, competence, self-regulation, and altruism as the core of medicine's professional status. George Lundberg (1990), a former editor of *JAMA*, considers professionalism to reside in self-governance, self-determination, and self-policing, adding that medicine has the responsibility to operate itself in the public interest.[8] Former Surgeon General C. Everett Koop, speaking about the declining sense of professionalism among physicians, notes that "the hallmark of a profession is that its members place the interests of those they serve above their own" (Koop, as quoted in Moore-West, Testa, and O'Donnell, 1998). Steven Schroeder, president of the Robert Wood Johnson Foundation, perceives professionalism as involving the core values of "service, compassion, and dedication" (1992). Frankford and Konrad (1998) define professionalism as a sense of commitment and control driven by a "deliberative process among equals," with the intrinsic value of work functioning as a key component of professionalism's normative vision. Hughes, Barker, and Reynolds (1994) define professionalism as a "set of values" (honesty and integrity), "attitudes" (humility and accountability to patients, colleagues, and society), and "behaviors" (being nonjudgmental and respectful to patients, pursuing specialized knowledge and skills, collegiality) that "results in serving the interests of patients and society before one's own." In their work developing a scale of professionalism, Arnold, Blank, Race, and Cipparone (1998) identify three components of professionalism: excellence, honor/integrity, and altruism/respect.[9] Finally, Wear (1997) highlights issues of compassion, social responsiveness, and reflectiveness in her work on professionalism. Wear also reminds us that the values of an organization are reflected in its organizational structure and its system of rewards, that the organizational structure of medicine (including medical training) is highly stratified, and that much of medical training is about attaching prerequisite values to the social and economic divisions of power located in these structures.

Countervailing Environments

Once again we must raise the troubling question of where within the process and practice of educating physicians are we to encounter pedagogical practices designed to enculturate these values and normative orientations. Whatever our responses, be they at the level of role models or clerkship evaluation forms, it is imperative to acknowledge that much of the value climate encountered by medical trainees is anything but neutral in tone or content. Sociologists (Becker, Geer, Hughes, & Strauss, 1961; Bloom, 1963; Bosk, 1979, 1992; Coombs, Chopra, Schenk, & Yutan, 1993; Hafferty, 1991; Leiderman & Grisso, 1985; Light, 1980; Merton, Reader, & Kendall, 1957; Mizrahi, 1986), anthropologists (Good & Good, 1989; Good, 1994; Konner, 1987), and medical insiders via accounts of the medical training process that are autobiographical (Cato 6, 1982; Doctor X, 1965; Hoffmann, 1990; Marion, 1989, 1991, 1998; Mullan, 1976) and quasi-autobiographical (Shem, 1978) have long documented the fundamentally moral nature of medical training. Within a related body of literature, medical students are depicted as constantly internalizing a variety of moral messages about the "rightness" and "wrongness" of various behaviors and attitudes as defined within the culture of medicine. Most of these messages, in turn, are delivered within the hidden and informal rather than the formal curriculum (Haas & Shaffir, 1982b; Hafferty, 1998; Hafferty & Franks, 1994; Hundert, 1997; Hundert, Douglas-Steele, & Bickel, 1996; Stern, 1996; Wallace, 1997; Wear, 1997).

In many respects, the values being transmitted within the hidden and informal curriculum are decidedly "unprofessional" in nature. For example, based on their work with undergraduates and residents, Feudtner and Christakis (1993) and Feudtner, Christakis, and Christakis (1994) found that medical students are routinely exposed to a range of deleterious influences, including the use of derogatory language by physicians when referring to patients and the falsification of patient records, along with unethical behaviors either their own and/or those of other members of their medical team. Almost two-thirds of their study respondents thought that their ethical principles had eroded because of their clinical experiences. In a second study (Christakis & Feudtner, 1997), the authors explored the ethical implications of physician-patient and physician-peer in-

Frederic W. Hafferty

teractions, the vast majority of which were "fleeting" in nature. Because of these transitory interactions, residents came to place a high value on "diagnostic cunning," gaming the system, and the delivery of care that was expediency- and discharge-oriented. The values of obligation and responsibility were marginalized. The authors concluded that "medicentric" values and procedures dominated residents' value systems. Work by DeWitt Baldwin and colleagues has uncovered a similar litany of transgressions, including falsification of patient records, sexual misconduct, physicians' delivery of care while impaired, cheating in research, and the cover-up of unethical behaviors and patient mistreatment (Baldwin, Daugherty, & Rowley, 1998; Sheehan, Sheehan, White, Leibovitz, & Baldwin, 1990). Extensive work by Self and colleagues documents that medical training inhibits or even undercuts the development of moral reasoning by medical students (Morton, Lamberton, Testerman, Worthley, & Loo, 1996; Self, Olivarez, & Baldwin, 1998; Self, Wolinsky, Baldwin, & Nease, 1989). In his study of residency training, Duncan (1996; also see Rainey, 1997) routinely witnessed sleep-deprived residents being called upon to carry out patient procedures they were ill trained to perform, inadequate supervision by attendings, and "needless" suffering by patients so that residents could learn.[10] Meanwhile, Shreves and Moss (1996) and Cohen (1999b) report that residents and attendings hold vastly different views on what constitutes an ethical problem or issue. Buttressing all these findings are additional studies that document a high prevalence of mistakes in clinical practice, most of which are unreported and "invisible" to the general public (Brennan et al., 1991; Davis, 1998; Hampson, 1995).

The clinic is not the only site of moral turpitude. Goe, Merrera, and Mower (1998) found a high level of applicants to medical school faculty positions provided false and incorrect information regarding their qualifications. Sekas and Hutson (1995) found misrepresentation of academic accomplishments by applicants for fellowship training. Meanwhile, both the scientific and public media routinely (it appears) report on health care fraud (e.g., Anders & McGinley, 1997; Eisler & Pearson, 1999), the falsification of scientific data (Hilts, 1991), and the incursion of the profit motive into academic (Cwiklik, 1998) and biomedical research (Langreth, 1998; Tanouye, 1998a, 1998b; Weber, 1998).

Finally, we need to acknowledge that medical students appear far more decisive than faculty and administration on how best to approach the "value conundrum." When offered coursework in professional skills and perspectives, medical students, almost universally, label this material as "inferior" (i.e., soft, ambiguous, and more subjective) to their coursework in the basic sciences and therefore less worthy of their academic time and efforts (see Makoul et al., 1998).

Moreover, when faced with the prospect of being evaluated on their profession-alism, students will protest — and faculty will capitulate — under the seemingly irrefutable charge that such evaluations lack rigor and objectivity (Steele & Sus-man, 1998).

Restructuring Medical Education

What, then, are we to conclude from this broad array of data and information on professions and professionalism? On one level, the task appears to be rela-tively straightforward. Working with the above definitions, medical educators need to construct a meaningful bridge between value orientations (compassion, commitment, a sense of obligation and responsibility, a fiduciary orientation) and structural parameters (collegiality, self-regulation and self-criticism, tech-nical competence). If history is to be our judge, such an undertaking is more easily proposed than accomplished. Legions of studies and commissions dating from the turn of the century have uniformly called for the training of a more sensitive and compassionate physician (Christakis, 1995). Part of the problem is that medical educators have yet to acknowledge that medical training — as cur-rently configured — is more about the education of an occupational class com-monly referred to as "professionals" than it is about "professional education." From a sociological vantage point, the entire range of medical education — from undergraduate through CME, which includes related credentialing struc-tures — continues to function more like a "certification mill" than a site of purposeful organizational activities devoted to the training of a workforce of "medical professionals" (Daugherty, personal communication, 1999). Medicine has long been loath to identify its members as "unprofessional." Approximately 98.5 percent of all individuals admitted to medical school in the United States will eventually acquire a license to practice medicine, a figure constant since the 1970s (Ludmerer, 1985). The inverse category (1.5 percent) signals a wide array of "events" including death, disability, and changing family circumstances — fac-tors far removed from the specter of "unprofessionalism." [11] Similarly, formal disciplinary action is taken against less than 1 percent of physicians in the United States each year (Scutchfield, 1998). And even here, the revocation of one's li-cense to practice medicine is associated more clearly with activities deemed "il-legal" than "unprofessional." In a defining statement, the Council on Ethical and Judicial Affairs of the AMA has called upon medicine to abandon its "con-spiracy of silence" surrounding unprofessional behavior (see AMA Policy Com-pendium, 1997).

Frederic W. Hafferty

Where then do we begin? For one, credentialing entities, such as the LCME, need to respond in a more positive manner to this "crisis of professionalism." As noted above, basic inconsistencies remain between core operating documents such as "The Structure and Function of the Medical School" and *The Medical Education Database* (the former has been defined by the longtime accreditation "insider" Andrew Hunt [1991] as the "bible of the accreditation process"). In addition, the movement to establish a competency-based evaluation system is an admirable step but still encumbered. The AAMC's Medical Student Objectives Project (MSOP) Report, for example, identifies four core competencies: altruism, knowledge, skill, and dutifulness. Along with definitions, each competency is accompanied by a list of "objectives" detailing how that competency might be assessed. But these lists of measurement possibilities are strangely stilted. Altruism is accompanied by seven objectives. Three begin with the phrase "Knowledge of" or "An understanding of." Another one refers to behavior ("Compassionate treatment of . . ."). One appears to bridge behavior and values ("Manifesting [although the item doesn't use this word] honesty and integrity"). Only two appear to fall more cleanly in the attitudes and values camp ("A commitment to advocate . . ." and "The capacity to recognize limitations and a desire to improve"). In short, the AAMC initially has defined its principle "value" item (altruism) more with respect to knowledge or behavior than in terms of values. Again, we can see an aversion to measuring core professional attributes in terms of its core elements.

Serious attention also needs to be paid to the admissions process. For too long, the medical school admissions committee, as a locus of standards and moral gatekeeper, has been assigned the "burden" of being the sole arbiter of assessing character and of presenting faculty with students who are altruistic, trustworthy, kind, and sensitive. But no one is exactly sure how admissions committees accomplish this daunting task, thus rendering the process a sociological black box. What we do know is that admissions procedures continue to emphasize MCAT and GPA scores in the decision-making processes (see Emmett, 1995; Oransky & Savitz, 1998).

Similarly, we need to move beyond remedial efforts in the "classroom" that have centered largely on restructuring the formal curriculum. Over the past two decades, courses have been added, deleted, restructured, integrated, compressed, and "made more relevant to the experiences of students." Journals such as *Academic Medicine* are awash with descriptions of courses in humanism, community service, and moral reasoning. But, as detailed elsewhere (Hafferty, 1999), medical educators have been unable to document how changes within the formal curriculum have resulted in more virtuous future physicians. A recent editorial by Foster (1998) in *Academic Medicine* is telling in this regard, not because the piece detailed how a district court upheld the right of a medical school to pay close attention to issues of character and honesty within the admissions process, but because medical education's foremost journal felt it necessary to remind the entire medical education community of this fact.

But the major barrier to developing a system of medical education around the concept of professionalism is cultural in nature. Medical educators and sociologists alike have yet to offer concrete suggestions as to how medical schools can work constructively within their hidden and informal curriculum to implement a value-based educational system while at the same time overcoming the countervailing values that have long dominated the educational milieu. When I was a neophyte faculty member over twenty-five years ago, I became intrigued by a particular question circulating among my medical students. "Whom would you rather have as your physician?" they asked each other. "An insensitive and boorish physician who knows everything or a warm and fuzzy physician who knows nothing?" I was perturbed by this question for several reasons, its obviously rhetorical nature notwithstanding.

Twenty-five years later, I still hear students asking this question and I am still bothered, but for a different reason. The dichotomy remains artificial, but I have come to see the question's durability as a reflection of the tremendous tensions that are embedded in the training process, and therefore the question itself as an important part of medicine's oral culture. Nonetheless, if I could have my way, I would prefer it to be phrased differently. Instead, I would have students ask, "Whom would you rather have as your physician? A technically competent but questionably professional physician or one with high professional standards who is less technically competent?" I prefer this latter phrasing for several reasons. First, the dichotomy of technical competence versus emotional sensitivity is not what I would like to term a "foundational comparison." The object of medical education is not emotional sensitivity. It is professionalism. Sensitivity is a subset of professionalism, and a qualified subset at that. Second, the contrast of technical proficiency versus professionalism is more historically accurate than the technical proficiency/sensitivity dichotomy. One need not read any further than Mary Shelley's *Frankenstein* or H. G. Wells's *The Island of Doctor Moreau* to understand how the public in the latter half of the nineteenth century came to fear science and medicine. These were not fears and fascinations about medicine's technical prowess per se, but about the motives and principles of those who were now infused with this new esoteric knowledge. Third, in our current world of managed care, raw technical competence, particularly when it is configured on the individual practitioner's level, is not considered to be a compelling and "positive" attribute. The world of managed care is a world that is quickly being "normalized" via practice protocols, guidelines, and report cards. "Excellence," in turn, is being defined more by a "regression to the mean" than by any sense of being "outstanding."

In short, I prefer my rewording of the classic knowledgeable/sensitive dichotomy because it places professionalism, not technical competence, at the core of the question. Although professionalism certainly can be configured in terms of proxies such as "customer satisfaction" or "adherence to protocols," I consider it more faithfully operationalized when it is defined in terms of individual commitments to attributes like compassion, caring, and a fiduciary orientation. Professionalism implies obligation and commitment, and both entities are better viewed as residing within individuals than within organizations. Finally, and to reiterate a previous point, although false dichotomies remain both specious and rhetorical, it is important to recognize that they do reflect points of tension within a culture and therefore occupy an important role within the socialization process. They may not be constructive, but they are instructive.

So, what are the action steps? Obviously, medical educators need to place a more traditionally faithful concept of professionalism at the core of medicine's educational mission. This begins by rewriting mission statements so that they highlight professionalism as a value — and include statements about what it means to be a professional (the mission statement that opens this chapter is an example of one that is in need of reform). In addition, and allowing important and necessary differences among schools, these mission statements need to frame "technical competence" and "academic excellence" as subsets of professionalism, not as "stand-alone" values or goals, and most surely not as the principal goal of the educational enterprise. Jordan Cohen is right: "The key to valuing the profession *is* to profess its values" (Cohen, 1998c; emphasis mine). But Cohen's dictum is not a trivial call to arms. Medical educators need to take a conscious and deliberate look at what should be placed at the core of medicine. Should it be technical competence, the answer medicine has provided for the past fifty years, or will it be professionalism? Historically, medicine has approached professionalism as a second-order variable. Medicine's declining professional status stands as testimony to the consequences of that decision. As we are reminded by Frankford and Konrad (1998), Southon and Braithwaite (1998), and others, professionalism *does* require a high level of technical expertise, but it does so *within* a core of professionalism, within a notion of commitment in which commitment stands as an end rather than as a means. Stated somewhat differently, the "perks" of professionalism, such as dominance, autonomy, power, and prestige, must function in the service of something else —

the role of the healer, for example (Cruess & Cruess, 1997). Operationally, this means that when mission statements are rewritten, faculty, students, and administration (in concert) must deliberately place professionalism at the apogee of their educational endeavors. Otherwise, "business as usual" will prevail, and notions of professionalism, if they are addressed at all, will be buried under the manifest task of preparing technically competent physicians.

Second, and to accomplish the above, medical educators, administrators, faculty, and students must acquire a better handle on the hidden and informal curriculum that exist within their learning environments. This means, among other things, that medical schools need to be approached as cultural entities and that change needs to be undertaken within a framework of the organization as a cultural system. There are a variety of strategies one can employ to this end (see Schein, 1992), so none will be detailed here, save to point out that remedial efforts will not be successful if they are carried out exclusively within the formal curriculum.

Third, medical educators need to explore ways to highlight service and the notion of medicine as a service-oriented occupation. One model, detailed by Eckenfels (1997), emphasizes the value of community experiences organized and run by students themselves. It is here, Eckenfels argues, that the values of service and a fiduciary orientation are internalized most successfully. For the most part, however, these types of curricular experiences remain in the control of faculty and administrators, are elective and selected by those who least "need" them, and thus stand as isolated islands of "authenticity" (Eckenfels, 1997) in a sea of egotism and entitlement (Dubovsky, 1987; Hundert et al., 1996). An analogous model described by Eckenfels exists in the U.S. Schweitzer Fellows Program (Forrow & Wolf, 1998). Organized around the belief that medical students "are hungry for opportunities to act on the ideals that brought them into [medicine]" and yet are "distracted" from the ideal of service by the educational system itself, the current Schweitzer program melds public service projects and personal reflection to "alter the culture of health professions schools in the direction of more meaningful cooperation with the surrounding community." Initially implemented in 1991, the program enrolls over one hundred new fellows each year.

Fourth, and most important, medical educators need to better understand the role of reflectiveness in the development and nurturance of professionalism. As we look back over the definitions of professionalism detailed above, there is an underlying yet undeniable message that the very nature of professional work (including the presence of uncertainty and the need for peer review) requires an ability by those who engage in professional work to step outside their own roles and norms and assume the position and place of "the other." It follows then, that medical students, as professionals-to-be, need to be afforded genuine learning opportunities in this respect. Calls for developing the reflective skills of medical students appear directly (see Frankford & Konrad, 1998; Lundberg, 1991; Wear, 1997) and indirectly, usually within broader discussions about themes of autonomy and self-regulation. In either case, what is being called for is a profound shift in value orientations — specifically the ability of physicians to better relate to the "other" which, not incidentally, constitutes the fundamental object of their work. But, as I detailed in my study of the emotional socialization of medical students (1991) and in writings on the hidden curriculum (Hafferty, 1999; Hafferty & Franks, 1994), the culture of medical training is infused with messages instructing students *not* to reflect "too much" on what is happening around them. These messages also include warnings about the "cost" of doing so, often framed in terms of a loss of technical knowledge. When approached from this vantage point, socialization can be understood as a process of internalizing norms and values about *not* reflecting on medical work, about *not* thinking too much about certain medical practices. In this same vein, writers such as Coles (1998), McEntyre (1997), and Gordon (1997) remind us that students' self-assessment skills are weak and not improved by conventional medical training. Coles (1998), for example, worries about the degree to which medical education functions as the "stifling of the moral imagination." Correspondingly, McEntyre (1997) characterizes medical education as a process of "de-familiarizing the familiar." In her autobiography of undergraduate medical training, Perri Klass (1987) expresses concern that she will be changed unwittingly and thus become "too hardened" or cynical. Autobiographical accounts of medical training are rife with examples of students unwittingly learning not to become too "caught up" in thinking about or "trying to make sense of" what is happening around them (Konner, 1987; Reilly, 1987; see also Conrad, 1988). The fourth law of Samuel Shem's "Laws of the House of God," "The patient is the one with the disease," is a wonderfully concise example of this normative dictate. These autobiographical tomes also illustrate the extent to which medical education involves a shroud of "mutual concealment" and a generalized "conspiracy of silence" (Conrad, 1988; Fox, 1988; Hafferty, 1991; Konner, 1987; Light, 1980). Even the dimension of time is transformed during medical training, and with considerable impact on the internalization of medicine's moral order (Christakis & Feudtner, 1997; Hafferty, 1991). In a world where the past often comes to reach back no further than the last exam, or when encounters with patients and peers are transient and evanescent, one should not be surprised to find medical trainees residing (often unwittingly) in an ever expanding (and nonreflective) here and now. Finally, the traditional emphasis on "technique" within the culture of medicine, embodied in the classic "the patient died but the operation was a success," elevates method over all other considerations and thus encourages the substitution of a narrow morality of technique for the more complex lay moral order (Bosk, 1979; Light, 1980).

The need is clear. Medical students — as future professionals — need to reflect upon the self and the relationship of the self to others. This requires, to invoke an old sociological phrase, the ability to stand in the other's shoes and to see oneself through the eyes of the other. This is not the equivalent of a "customer is always right" mentality. It does mean, however, that the physician should possess the value orientations and the necessary skills to acknowledge meaningfully the place of the other in the provision of medical services. If the self is not to be a part of the therapeutic encounter then all the above is superfluous, and we are talking about the delivery of medicine by technicians — not professionals.

The manner in which all this is to be accomplished remains elusive. To date, the principal vehicles identified in the medical education literature are humanities courses in which literature (poetry, fiction, autobiography) is reviewed and discussed with the hope that students will learn to "experience" medicine from a variety of perspectives (Hunter, Charon, & Coulehan, 1995; Moore-West, Testa, & O'Donnell, 1998). Once again, these courses usually are elective and most often attended by "the choir." Those most in need, however, remain aloof in their disdain. Perhaps most disconcerting, as detailed by Moore-West, Testa, and O'Donnell (1998), "insight" is an elusive commodity that sometimes comes at the cost of student anger, resentment, and, parenthetically, negative course evaluations.

Critics may argue that I am being too harsh on medical education and that much is being done to establish, maintain, and even enhance professionalism during medical training. I disagree. In doing so, I offer the following litmus test. The most valid way to ascertain what medical schools truly value is to scrutinize the premed advisement students receive in college along with the products offered by MCAT and USMLE National Board preparation industry (Hafferty, 1999). If medical schools truly are serious about recruiting and training sensitive, ethical, and service-oriented physicians, then I would expect that Kaplan Educational Centers, Princeton Review, and similar companies would be providing "training in" or "exposures to" these types of attributes and experiences. But they do not. Correspondingly, if medical schools truly are serious about recruiting and training sensitive, ethical, and service-oriented physicians, then medical school hopefuls would demand that Kaplan and Princeton provide them with the necessary edge in these areas. In response to this "new market," companies like Kaplan would allocate considerable resources to developing, advertising, and marketing these "necessary" products and services. In turn, medical school hopefuls would spend the millions of dollars they now devote to acquiring a technically based expertise on acquiring a "high professionalism" profile instead. All this — mission statements, formal and hidden curricula, services, advertising, and consumer demand (and fear) — would constitute a new social construction of reality (Berger & Luckman, 1966), thus underwriting the new professionalism medicine says it so desperately seeks. However, to reiterate an earlier point, *we* are not the necessary object of persuasion about medicine's commitment to professionalism. "Stanley Kaplan" is. And until I see Kaplan and others offering such services, I will continue to conclude that medical schools have not placed professionalism at the core of their mission.

As we witness the rise of the corporation and the commodification of medical services, we find ourselves coming full circle — sociologically speaking. Where Durkheim and others considered the rise of a professional class to be a necessary and important response to the growth of industrialization, others, a century later, are beginning to call on professionalism in response to the rise of a corporate and governmental presence in the organization and delivery of medical services. These more recent calls for professionalism are more limited than those of a century ago. For Durkheim, the professional was a buffer between the state / corporation and the masses. Durkheim did not restrict his analysis to issues of health and medicine. While it is understandable that we harbor concerns about a culture of commercialism within medicine, it is important to recognize that medicine's ills are but a small piece of a much larger social transformation. It is not "the doctor" who is under attack. It is the professional. The danger is not "alternative medicine" or "complementary providers" but the rise of the technician. Durkheim envisioned the professional as a servant of the masses and professionalism as a process of work geared toward solving complex social problems. We should adopt the same broad frame of reference.

NOTES

1. For an article to be counted as "highlighting issues of medicine as professionalism," some form of the word "professional" needed to appear in the title, the abstract, or a major section heading within the body of the paper.

2. A "reverse count" of articles in which issues of professionalism might have appeared but did not (e.g., the future of academic health centers and medical education in an era of managed care) would have been equally illuminating, but was not undertaken.

3. For an exception, see the "Profession of Medicine Program" (POMP) at the University of Wisconsin (Swick & Simpson, 1998).

4. Hensel and Dickey (1998) note that, in an "ideal world," the phrase "ethical professional" would be redundant because "one must be ethical to be a professional."

5. Raelin (1986) defines the conflict more broadly as being a cultural clash between "managers" and professionals.

6. More specifically, Swick (1998, p. 752) contrasts the "major capitalistic values" of profit, competition, responsibility to stockholders, services driven by the market, standards set by external forces, consumerism, short-term goals, and giving society what it thinks it wants, with the "major values of the medical profession" (service, advocacy, altruism, services driven by the application of a specialized body of knowledge, standards set and maintained internally, humanism, long-term goals, and meeting society's needs).

7. The study drew its data from the 125 US medical schools, four focus groups of managed care practitioners, administrators, educators, and residents, and a national sample of physicians and medical directors (Meyer, Potter, & Gary, 1997).

8. In a second editorial (1991), Lundberg advocated that "the essence of professionalism is self-governance. Central to self-governance is self-criticism."

9. In their scale, the excellence factor loaded items of role models and modeling and altruism. The honor/integrity item tapped issues related to falsification of patient records and lying. The altruism/respect item touched upon references to patients or other health care workers in a derogatory manner and organization of work for convenience rather than for the patient (Arnold, Blank, Race, & Cipparone, 1998).

10. The notions of medical training as "stressful" or "abusive" are open to considerable discussion. Counts of abuse, for example, include reports of "unfair grades" (Hafferty, 1999), while levels of stress among medical students, when measured using externally validated instruments, may be considerably less than what is concluded to be the case based on more descriptive kinds of data (see Toews et al., 1997).

11. This is not to say that students do not fail courses or that the approximately 5 percent USMLE failure rate is not viewed with apprehension and fear by those taking the national boards. Still, virtually all students failing exams, be they school based or national, eventually will acquire a license to practice medicine.

Frederic W. Hafferty

RICHARD MARTINEZ

Professional Role in Health Care Institutions
Toward an Ethics of Authenticity

The growing interest in the concept of professionalism in health care education is welcomed by many of us who teach and work in health care institutions. In recent years, many health care education journals have featured articles on some aspect of professionalism. However, the concept of professionalism, like pornography, can be elusive when considered in the real world of patient care and medical education. Models of health care professionalism that invoke the Hippocratic and related traditions are argued as a standard. Often, this standard is used to judge other models wherein professionalism is determined solely by current social needs and desires, detached from the historical traditions of the profession. This latter view, where the social construction of values trumps the tradition and history of a profession, can add to the confusion over many of our current professional dilemmas in health care. In addition, questions about the proper relationship between the medical and business aspects of health care practice are on the rise as health care professionals and health care institutions adjust to changes in reimbursement practices. Translating the concept of professionalism into educational materials and experiences can be difficult.

The gap between the values of health care professionals and health care institutional priorities is widening. In health professional educational institutions, including medical schools, this is of tremendous concern. In this chapter, I discuss the problem of individual responsibility in the face of conflict with institutional values and goals. As Elizabeth Wolgast notes in her book *Ethics of an Artificial Person: Lost Responsibility in Professions and Organizations* (1992), many of our modern professions and organizations diffuse and discourage individual responsibility by promoting the phenomenon of individual persons speaking and acting in the name of the group. In many health care institutions, including our medical schools and teaching hospitals, professional identity and the responsibilities coupled to that identity are conceptualized as the professional role. I consider the concept of professional role to be a significant contributor to the worrisome trend of diffusing individual responsibility in the name of institutional and organizational priorities.

In the health care professions, as in other professions, the places where many professionals work and learn are large and impersonal institutions. In such places, conflicts between the values of individuals and institutional priorities are common. In health care education, too often, health care professionals and students feel powerless to resolve these conflicts in a direction that fosters individual personal and professional integrity. When professional role is considered primarily in the narrow sense of social role, individual moral conflict that emerges in working and training in institutions and organizations can be marginalized. This leaves many professionals and students with feelings of powerlessness, and, too often, morally traumatized. Unfortunately, institutional priorities in this age of health care reform often support narrow views of professional role whereby individuals are seen as extensions of institutional priorities. This then discourages authentic individual moral expression, especially when conflict arises between institutions and individuals.

The Silencing of Institutional Critics

In the managed care climate, many of our health care institutions discourage individual professionals and students from expressing views or taking actions that might disrupt the priorities and goals of those institutions. "Gag clauses" in contracts between physicians and managed care organizations stand as dramatic examples of this reality in recent times. "Noncompete clauses" are not uncommon in the contractual arrangements between professionals and the health care institutions that employ them. Medical students who complain about curricular priorities or become advocates for particular patients can be dismissed as "complainers." These arrangements and attitudes can silence professionals and students, making criticism of institutional priorities unlikely. In health care institutions, including medical educational institutions, the trend toward valuing professionals and students instrumentally seems to be on the rise, contributing to the growing numbers of discouraged and unhappy health care professionals. The moral and practical effects of this trend on patient care are only beginning to be appreciated.

As with individuals, contradictions occur between the stated values and the actual behavior of institutions. However, educators must encourage identifica-

Richard Martinez

tion and critical analysis of these ethical lapses if we are to reverse certain emerging and alarming trends familiar to many of us who teach and work in health care institutions. It is common to see individual "critics" as "complainers," rarely supported and valued, often viewed as undesirable and dispensable. This is particularly worrisome in our medical schools and university-affiliated hospitals, where patient care is at stake.

Engaging faculty and students in critical examination of societal and cultural problems, supporting and rewarding professional ideals and independent expression, and encouraging ethical reflection and deliberation upon institutional goals and values are necessary activities for positive institutional change. Criticism, whether by individuals or through programmatic elements such as ethics committees and humanities curricular developments, is necessary if we are serious about creating healthy institutions where ethical practices matter. Yet current concepts of professional role in health care education do not include the activities and values necessary to support institutional critics. Compliance with institutional goals and priorities is valued over the identification and critical analysis of institutional moral failures. Increasingly, professional role responsibilities are defined in narrow terms that support institutional goals and discourage critical perspective. Furthermore, in this time of health care reform, it is increasingly the case that institutional priorities conflict with the goals of patients, health care professionals, and health care professional students.

Promoting a professional identity situated primarily in the concept of professional role poses problems and dangers in medical education. How does the concept of professional role contribute to the diffusion of personal responsibility in the medical setting, while silencing the critical voices necessary for the development of moral institutional practices? How does professional role limit and obfuscate the proper place of personal values and beliefs in the individual professional's life and decisions? Is there a place for professional and personal integrity in the concept of role? How does the medical educational process encourage the creation of "artificial persons" speaking and acting for the institution and its values, while discouraging the development of authentic persons who are free to identify, criticize, and challenge institutional practices and goals? These considerations are important when we consider the enculturation process by which health care professional students begin to internalize the values of teachers and mentors, as well as those of the institutions where they work and learn. The processes by which institutions and organizations undermine personal responsibility is most disturbing when we understand the impact this can have on patients and their families.

Professional Role, Boundaries, and Role Morality

F. H. Bradley, the nineteenth-century British idealist who attempted to locate the source of morality in the consciousness of individuals and institutions of his time, argued that "self-realization" occurs when duty and happiness are joined: "Yes, we have found ourselves, when we have found our station and its duties, our function as an organ in the social organism" (Bradley, 1988, p. 163). Bradley, like Hegel before him, reacted to the Kantian moral absolutes by locating morality, both common morality and role morality, in cultural and historical particulars. Influenced by the class distinctions and social hierarchical constraints of his day, Bradley is often cited as the source of current role morality theory, where moral behavior is located in the role obligations defined by our place in the social order.

Roles are sometimes considered through the metaphor of theater. In roles, as with players in a dramatic production, masks and costumes can be worn to cover a true self. In our professions, we are similarly players in a theatrical performance, where the stage, the script of the play, and the director influence the extension and limit of our actions. However, as players we cannot help but bring ourselves, our natural selves, to our performance. Our unique interpretation of the playwright's script, the way we move across the stage, the holding of the head, the look in our eyes, the manner of gesturing with our hands, the cadence and particulars of speech — all of these reflect the uniqueness of the person behind the assigned character in the play. And so it is with professional roles, both constrained by professional obligations and responsibilities, and yet open to the possibility of the natural and unique person expressing herself through the playing of her part.

However, as the analogy suggests, one can only go so far in the expression of that uniqueness before the character in the play is no longer represented, or before we say that this is the worst performance of *King Lear* we have ever seen. There are limits to allowing personal qualities to find expression in the role one is playing. With professional roles, there are limits beyond which most professionals are reluctant to tread, for fear that they are no longer conducting themselves as professionals and may actually harm patients. Maintaining a role, in this sense, is useful and helpful. In situations where professional role and the institutional structure that contains (or constrains) one in a role are united in moral priorities, the concept of professional role is adequate in delineating individual responsibility.

What happens when institutions and individuals are not united in moral pri-

Richard Martinez

orities? How does professional role serve both the institution and the individual in the role? A narrow sense of professional role, that is, defined primarily as a social role, is inadequate when conflicts occur between institutions and individuals. Indeed, within this narrow sense of role, one's experience of functioning primarily in a socially determined professional role can result in the diffusion of personal responsibility. Unfortunately, failures to respond in humane and compassionate ways to patients are often justified by a narrow understanding of one's professional role: "I was only a third-year medical student: I didn't think I should give the patient a Kleenex since no one else in the ER did." One medical student told me this in describing his guilt after failing to respond to a crying woman whose son required abdominal surgery following an automobile accident. The student believed that to comfort a crying patient "is not part of the job description for ER docs."

Elizabeth Wolgast traces the concept of "artificial," "feigned," or "fictional" persons to Thomas Hobbes, who introduced the concept to explain the relationship between citizens and representative government speaking on their behalf. Using examples such as servants acting for their employers and parents deciding for their children in identifying the concept of "artificial" persons, Hobbes ignored the problem of moral agency involved in such relationships. Wolgast picks up Hobbes's "artificial persons" and provides a thoughtful and complex analysis of the problem of moral agency in modern institutions. Concerned about the diffusion of individual responsibility in modern professions and organizations, she states that modern institutions must seek reform. "The motive for tackling these gargantuan projects of reform, however, is that the alternative is a further thinning in the meaning of responsibility on one side while nurturing institutions that defeat it on the other. A decision to change is acutely a moral decision, and moral courage is needed to make it" (Wolgast, 1992, p.157). Translated to medical education, we should support and encourage medical students, house officers, and faculty who speak of moral discomfort, supporting their "critical" speech and action within our medical schools and teaching hospitals.

Increasingly, the significance of professional role is linked to consideration of boundaries in the professional-patient relationship. Discussions of professional misconduct, for example, draw on the concept of boundaries: a broad consideration of boundary dilemmas would include, at one end of a continuum, a physician's sexual misconduct with patients, and at the other end, issues such as how to respond to gifts or whether to treat a family member for minor medical problems.

Conflicts in which the values of individual professionals or students are at odds with the priorities of the institutions in which they work and learn also involve boundaries. What is the proper relationship between these individuals and institutional goals? What boundary dilemmas characterize this relationship? As in the professional-patient relationship, the relationship between individuals and institutions requires trust, communication, free exchange of information, and avoidance of coercion and exploitation.

The concept of professional role is argued as a means of managing boundaries. Interpreted broadly, with room for flexibility and individual exceptions, it protects both the professional and the patient. While there are obvious differences between the intensity of the relationships of the professional involved in weekly psychotherapy and his/her anxious patient and the family physician who sees a patient twice in a year for elevated cholesterol, a view of role applied narrowly, in either case, can lead to both patient injury and damage to the relationship. In other words, rigid adherence to the prohibition against boundary crossings and dual relationships, joined to a narrow view of professional role, limits aspiration toward and the cultivation of professional ideals. The ideal of a moral, healing, humane experience with one's patient is excluded when one is narrowly involved in the experience of professional role.

Drawing on these concepts of boundaries and professional role, we can better understand the relationship between the individual and the health care institutions where we work and learn together. If we wish to support moral ideals, the boundary between institutions and individuals must become flexible, encourage communication and trust, and avoid coercion. Professionals must be regarded as unique individuals, not "artificial persons" who speak and act only on behalf of the institution. Innovation, creativity, and open communication must be valued in the dynamics between individuals and the organizations.

————

In the following examples of boundary problems, two trainees, T. J. and M. K., are faced with situations in which the potential for harming their respective patients is clear. Both situations involve persons in authority modeling behaviors that trouble trainees. In both situations, the trainees are uncomfortable with the possibility of confronting those authority figures. The dynamics of professional role, situated in the hierarchical reality of medical education and practice, are illustrated here.

T. J. is thirty years old and a fourth-year medical student. While on a clinical medicine rotation at a large teaching hospital, he approached his supervising chief resident, and expressed the desire to practice certain elements of the physical exam of which he had yet to develop full mastery. Two weeks into his rotation, while spending an afternoon in the medical outpatient clinic, the chief resident told him to join another resident, Dr. D. S. in room 10 to "perform a rectal," and "practice the examination of the prostate." T. J. knocked on the door of room 10.

A voice from behind the closed door shouted to come in and close the door. Upon entering, T. J. saw a white male, approximately fifty years old, his back to Dr. D. S., bending over an examination table, his pants and underwear dropped to his ankles. The resident, Dr. D. S., without introducing T. J. to the patient or himself to T. J., told T. J. to "get a glove on and lube up." As T. J. pulled on a glove and lubricated it, Dr. D. S., in a "gruff voice," told the unidentified patient that T. J. was going to perform a "rectal exam," and added, "This won't hurt." The patient dutifully assumed the appropriate position for the exam. As Dr. D. S. guided T. J.'s hand and finger in the exam, the patient groaned in discomfort. Neither Dr. D. S. or T. J. comforted the patient, but continued with the "practice exam."

Several weeks later, T. J. reported that he was ashamed for not interrupting the procedure when the patient expressed discomfort. Furthermore, he expressed his confusion over his failure to introduce himself to the patient before the exam, even though Dr. D. S. had also ignored this common courtesy. T. J. described himself as "being caught in a whirlwind." He said, "I felt it happened so fast that I wasn't sure what was the right thing to do. I was afraid of offending the resident." T. J. also expressed concern about complaining, saying he felt that "this goes on all the time" in medical training, and he was fearful that he would be seen by other medical students and his supervisors as a "complainer."

———

M. K. is thirty-two years old and in pursuit of a second career after working for years as a flight attendant. She is a nursing student who works in a pediatric intensive care unit in a large teaching hospital. She was involved in the care of a three-year-old patient who, after a ten-day hospitalization in the ICU, had died. M. K. had developed a relationship with the parents over the ten days, and directed them from the waiting room to a cubicle within the ICU, placing the dead child in the mother's arms.

While sitting with the family, she heard, from the other side of the curtain, several voices engaged in a discussion "about finances and the stock market." She recognized one of these voices as that of a senior physician who was routinely involved in the care of children in the ICU, although not the dead child's care. With some anxiety, M. K. apologized to the family, walked to the nursing station, and asked the senior physician and two other physicians to lower their voices. She told them of the death of the child and of the child's parents in the nearby cubicle. The physicians complied without protest or annoyance. They were apologetic.

M. K. later reported feeling frightened and uncomfortable in approaching these senior physicians. "I was afraid they would be annoyed with me. All three physicians are supervisors and have much power. I knew I would be working with them again, and that they might have input into my evaluation."

––––––––

The literature in medical education is replete with descriptions of the enculturation process where values are modeled, certain behaviors are rewarded, and others discouraged. In the examples of T. J. and M. K., we are reminded of this enculturation process. Rigid institutionalized roles and obedience to already existing hierarchical structures within institutions stabilize power dynamics and promote efficiency. Mechanisms such as ethics committees, construed to support and encourage reflection upon the institution's ethical domain, may be looked upon with suspicion, since their processes might require change in curricular priorities and clinical practices, and the redistribution of limited resources. A view of professional role that includes the responsibilities of identifying and criticizing institutional moral failure would require changes in health care education. Just as flexibility and the cultivation of professional ideals in the patient-professional relationship are advantageous, so a more courageous professional role and more flexible boundaries in the relationship between institutions and the individuals training and working in these institutions are desirable. Encouragement and support for critical voices are necessary if we are to create educational environments that promote ethical ideals.

In the first example, T. J.'s "whirlwind" is his metaphor for the automatic and often unconscious manner in which young medical students are brought in line with role expectations. T. J. walks into a room where a patient is in a vulnerable position. The resident, who is modeling behavior for T. J., fails to introduce the patient and behaves in a manner in which both the patient and T. J. are transformed from human beings to instruments of the institution. The patient is reduced to the function of providing an "educational experience" for T. J., while T. J. performs the role of obedient fourth-year medical student in need of that "experience." The resident fulfills his institutional role, following instructions from his supervising chief resident, by bringing the two together to further the goals of the medical school. That is, T. J. and the patient are reduced to objects who participate as if "caught in a whirlwind" toward the pragmatic institutional goal of providing future physicians for society.

Regrettably, this situation is not uncommon in our medical schools and teaching hospitals. Failure to recognize and remedy harm to both patients and participating professionals and students is commonplace. Given institutional priorities, the hierarchical elements of medical training, the ease with which "educational experiences" take precedence over moral considerations, and the particular pressures felt by this medical student to conform and obey, a more humane and respectful experience for those involved was unlikely. The medical student, his resident supervisors, and the patient, through the automatic and unconscious assumption of professional roles and patient roles, colluded with and supported the goals of the institution. Furthermore, because there are no legitimate ways for this student to acknowledge and criticize this experience, the institution remains unaware of its moral failure.

In M. K.'s situation, the power relationship between nurses and physicians plays a significant role. M. K., a nursing student not yet confident of her relationship to other health care professionals, felt uncomfortable about the physicians' conversation near the area where she was comforting grieving parents. The juxtaposition of images is dramatic. Grieving parents have watched their child die, and a compassionate nursing student attempts to provide comfort. Out of sight but within earshot, three physicians discuss the subject that supports our worst impressions about professionals in our society — money. Fortunately, by confronting the three physicians, M. K. was able to transcend a narrow professional role, one in which students "take orders" from supervisors and where obedience and compliance are highly valued. In most discussions of professional role, a broad view that considers individual professional aspirations toward moral ideals is neglected. In M. K.'s account, we see the importance of personal values and professional integrity in determining her decent and courageous action. We learn of her personal conflict with her presumed role when she speaks of her discomfort at confronting the three physicians. Fortunately, she transcends this presumed role, and acts independently. Her view is of a professional role that requires integrity and loyalty to one's personal morality. M. K. exercises her individual sense of decency and respect for patients.

Authenticity and Integrity

Charles Taylor (1991) argues for an "ethics of authenticity" in postmodern life. He describes the three "malaises," or cultural declines, of our time: first, excessive individualism that has replaced social commitment and common societal values; second, dominance of instrumental reason in our individual and collective lives; and, third, the restriction of choice fostered by the institutions and structures of industrial-technological society. He also describes two common responses to these malaises. The "knockers" are those who see only terrible moral decline, narcissism, loss of individual choice to the technological victory, and nihilism. The "boosters" are those who believe that the idea of personal freedom is overblown and that scientific progress is intrinsically good in its improvement of material life. Rather than choose between the "knockers" and the "boosters" of this postmodern predicament, Taylor argues for a moratorium on cultural pessimism, even as he delineates the potential dangers and opportunities of our times. We are reminded of Søren Kierkegaard when he argues that

> each one of us has an original way of being human [and that] entails that each of us has to discover what it is to be ourselves. But the discovery can't be made by consulting pre-existing models, by hypothesis. So it can be made only by articulating it afresh. We discover what we have it in us to be by becoming that mode of life, by giving expression in our speech and action to what is original in us. The notion that revelation comes through expression is what I want to capture in speaking of the "expressivism" of the modern notion of the individual. (Taylor, 1991, p. 61)

Taylor's view of authenticity is of a moral ideal. As with Lionel Trilling before him, Taylor believes that authenticity involves being "true to oneself," not simply self-interested, or engaged in narcissistic self-fulfillment. "What do I mean by a moral ideal?" Taylor asks. "I mean a picture of what a better or higher life would be, where 'better' and 'higher' are defined not in terms of what we happen to desire or need, but offer a standard of what we ought to desire" (1991, p. 16). Such a view is an antidote to the narrow concept of professional role that serves institutional purposes and defines professional identity in much of contemporary life. An ethics of authenticity in our institutions of medical education demands a place for the "expressivism" of individuals within these institutions. Critics of institutional values and goals must be encouraged, not banished. Abandoning narrow views of professional role and mechanical notions of boundaries will go far in creating better relationships between institutions and their dependents.

———

Boundary dilemmas — the tension between personal and professional morality — can tell us much about the nature of professionalism. An article by Miller and Brody (1995) offers a view of professional integrity relevant to this discussion. The authors begin by defining personal integrity as a dimension of identity, involving activities that cultivate or harm trust, and that reflect qualities of wholeness and intactness. For the individual, three elements are necessary for integrity:

Richard Martinez

a set of well-regarded values and principles that remain somewhat stable over time and are coherent; verbal expression of those values and principles; and consistency between what one says and what one does. Overrigid adherence to values and principles and inflexibility in conduct are not regarded as aspects of integrity.

Whereas personal integrity is closely connected to individual identity, according to Miller and Brody, professional identity and professional integrity are more socially determined, as is the case with professional role in general. While in the role of professional, the individual acts in accordance with community-defined expectations and restrictions on individual expression. Here we see elements of Bradley's "my station and its duties." However, the concept of professional integrity is more robust than the professional role thus far discussed — that is, the view of professional role primarily determined by social expectations. Professional integrity provides a more dynamic understanding of the interplay of personal and professional morality. More important, professional integrity supports individual expression in those situations where institutional priorities and goals are in conflict with individual values. "Professional role," as a sociological concept, tends to conjoin the values of the institution and the individual. When there is conflict, the concept of professional role steers the moral equation toward the priorities of the institution. If, within a concept of professional integrity, there is conflict, support for the thoughtful, even critical individual and her values is favored.

All professions maintain an internal set of goals, duties, values, and ideals that are essential for professional identity and integrity. If these internal standards are abandoned, one might wear the trappings of that profession, but would no longer be a representative of the profession. In addition, individuals in all professions possess personal standards and values — a personal morality — that shape and influence their professional identity and integrity. In other words, individual personal morality influences professional morality. At the same time, the concept of professional role often marginalizes and diminishes the influence of these personal values in the actions of professionals. Whether we are physicians, teachers, or lawyers, our obligations to those we serve, whether derived from external codes and rules or from the profession's internal standards and norms, are influenced by personal morality. We cannot expunge from professional morality these individual personal values and beliefs. Nor is this desirable.

While good arguments are put forth for minimizing personal considerations in professional life, the danger of objectification of persons by our institutions through the concept of professional role requires a critical look. Once people become objects, instrumental values are likely to dominate in the exchanges between individuals and institutions. Ultimately, an ethos of instrumental values is fostered in such communities. In health care institutions, we cannot afford to treat individuals as mere means to instutional priorities. When such an ethos takes hold, not only are the individuals violated within our health care institutions, but the institutions are no longer serving the purpose for which they are intended. Medical schools and teaching hospitals are places for training health professionals, but their first priority is the care of sick, injured, and dying persons. When this care becomes simply a means to provide educational experiences for professional trainees and a laboratory for scientific inquiry, the moral rescue of the institution is doubtful. We need strong and critical individuals within our health care institutions to remind us of early evidence of moral breakdown.

Nazi doctors involved in institutional killing considered themselves physicians. Many argued that they were acting on behalf of the goals of the German state, turning their expertise and knowledge to that end. However, their behavior and the perverted values that drove it could not be considered a new role for physicians in "the Nazi community." Physicians who torture and kill are something other than physicians, if not according to the regime that supports such activity, then in the eyes of history. Robert Lifton (1986) describes a "doubling" phenomenon that allowed Nazi physicians to separate their personal morality from their professional role. In part, this phenomenon reflects a tenaciously held view that the physician is primarily a role, socially determined and unencumbered by personal morality.

The intrinsic values and the activities of professions define the profession. Just as personal integrity has a certain consistency over time, a profession possesses tradition and, according to Miller and Brody, a "historical narrative" of the goals, duties, values, and ideals of the profession. This historical narrative informs the role of the professional and anchors it, buffering it and the individual professional against the vagaries of social and situational forces. This is especially important when these forces place pressure on the professional to behave in a manner contrary to the historical narrative. Recent experience with "gag clauses" illustrates this point: Managed care organizations attempted to restrict communication between physicians and their patients about treatments and other interventions not offered in their medical plans. The historical narrative of the health professions supported the courage and professional integrity of a few individual critics (some were fired from the organizations who employed them), and has led to a national backlash against this destructive intrusion into the physician-patient relationship.

A narrow concept of professional role fails to mediate adequately the tension

Richard Martinez

between this historical narrative of the profession and the impact of personal morality in our professional decisions. Role morality and the concept of professional role are intended to reduce harm. However, just as rigid adherence to professional roles in therapeutic relationships can damage and harm patients, narrow views of professional role can undermine the integrity of both individuals and the institutions where health professionals work and are trained. By increasing allegiance to institutions while diminishing commitments to individual patients and to one's own personal morality, this narrow concept of professional role can diffuse and discourage individual responsibility. Medicine's historical narrative of its professional integrity requires and encourages a different kind of relationship between health care institutions and the individuals who work and train within those institutions.

––––––––

The question of the right thing to do for one's patient is coupled to the question of the kind of professional one is. Similarly, one's professionalism is inevitably affected by dynamic relationship between individual and institution. What professional values guide the individual professional? How does the institution support or discourage these values and ideals? Is the voice of the critic encouraged, or seen as a threat? What are the institution's values in the domain of individual expression? Does the institution support individuals in their struggle with personal and professional conflict? And finally, are professional roles defined narrowly, in terms that serve institutional goals, or broadly, in terms that support robust notions of professional integrity and authenticity and of boundaries that are to be explored, not rigidified?

Our profession is a large part of who we are, and it is deeply connected to the larger community that includes and supports us. In his book *Lawyers and Justice: An Ethical Study* (1988), David Luban provides insight into why we must ask questions about professionalism. He argues that "commitments to the duties of a profession, to a career, or to major social institutions . . . are among the deepest loyalties and commitments in our lives; and it cannot be right to ask us to reconsider them, to trade them off, again and again. A person who was willing to do this, we may think, is morally frightening, not commendable" (p. 142).

F. H. Bradley understood the limits of "my station and its duties" when he noted that the community "may be in a confused or rotten condition, so that in it right and might do not always go together" (Bradley, 1988, p. 203). Bradley argues, as I have, for the voice of the critic. We must challenge those institutions that ask us to behave in ways that are morally reprehensible, even if we sacrifice our personal comfort. Personal and professional integrity require it. In the words of Bradley, "We must wrap ourselves in a virtue which is our own and not the world's, or seek a higher doctrine by which, through faith and through faith alone, self-suppression issues in a higher self-realization. . . . You cannot confine a man to his station and its duties" (p. 204).

In medical education, the growing interest in professionalism is cause for some celebration. The economic, political, social, and cultural influences on the practice of health care are complex: this is a time of great uncertainty for professionals and students in health care. In this chapter, I have argued for a view of professionalism that is critical of restrictive concepts of professional roles. I argue now for the need to create and nurture institutional processes and mechanisms within our medical schools and teaching hospitals that welcome the voices of those who identify and criticize troublesome institutional goals, or the means by which institutions pursue legitimate goals.

These institutional processes can come in many shapes and forms: hospital ethics committees; curricular changes that encourage reflection on moral failure at the institutional level; the creation of legitimate and institutionally supported ethics "debriefing sessions" for students, staff, and residents; and the establishment of policies and procedures within our health care institutions that encourage and support proper avenues for the expression of "moral grievances." All such mechanisms for change must involve values and activities that cultivate and support trust, communication, and free exchange of information while guarding against coercion and exploitation in the relationship between individuals and institutions.

An "ethics of authenticity" requires that we support individual action and speech, even when they are critical of things we cherish. If institutions are to cultivate a healthy moral climate, this support must come from those who are privileged, and thus obligated and able to nurture. Medical educators and administrators must support institutional mechanisms whereby individual professionals and students can identify, criticize, and seek change in institutional processes and activities that compromise their moral integrity and, ultimately, the integrity of the institution itself.

Richard Martinez

JACK COULEHAN

PETER C. WILLIAMS

Professional Ethics and Social Activism

Where Have We Been? Where Are We Going?

When Andrea Fricchione visited Stony Brook for her medical school interview, she radiated warmth and enthusiasm. She had graduated with honors from a prestigious liberal arts college, but had purposely not applied directly to medical school. Instead, she chose to spend a year as a teacher with a volunteer organization in inner-city Baltimore. Like the vast majority of the seven hundred or so applicants we invite each year for interviews, Andrea had a snappy-looking "pre-med portfolio" that included excellent grades and test scores, considerable health-related volunteer experience, a wide array of undergraduate extracurricular activities, significant experience in a research laboratory, and a personal statement that described her compelling commitment to medicine. In addition, Andrea graduated with a humanities major.

What tipped the balance in favor of admitting Andrea? There were a number of factors. For one thing the faculty interviewer was quite impressed with her thoughtfulness and maturity. When asked about her emergency room volunteer work, Andrea could tell stories of her interactions with specific patients, rather than just making global statements about how meaningful the experience was. When asked what book she had read recently, Andrea described in detail both the book and her reaction to it. She was well informed about ethical and social issues in contemporary medicine. Andrea had been a leader in a number of organizations in college. In fact, she had organized an HIV-education project on campus and later served as a student member of her college's curriculum committee. Andrea's decision to devote a year to teaching underprivileged children was another plus — it helped prove that she not only had a strong sense of social commitment, but also the courage to act on it.

We were pleased when Andrea chose to attend Stony Brook over the other medical schools that accepted her. During her preclinical years, she became an active proponent (as well as a thoughtful critic) of Medicine in Contemporary Society (MCS), Stony Brook's four-year curriculum in the medical humanities and social issues in medicine. As a result of our confidence in her insight and candor, a couple of months before she graduated we asked Andrea to reflect in writing on her medical school experience, placing particular emphasis on issues of altruism and social consciousness. The following are excerpts from her statement:

"When I arrived in medical school, I was eager to get involved," Andrea wrote. "I was excited about addressing important issues because I was sure that, as medical students, we would have some clout and certainly a commitment to the well-being of others."

"However, medical school is an utter drain," she continued.

For two years lecturers parade up and down describing their own particular niche as if it were the most important thing for a student to learn. And then during the clinical years, life is brutal. People are rude, the hours are long, and there is always a test at the end of the rotation. . . . After a while I reasoned that the most important thing I could do for my patients, for my fellow human beings, for the future of medicine, as well as for me, was to assure myself some peaceful time. I made a point of hoarding my extra time for simple pleasures. I had read Perri Klass's novel in which she describes how physicians must relearn the ability to appreciate the mundane. Her point is that physicians must regain their humanity after completing their training. For my part, I tried not to lose it, or at least to hold onto it as long as possible. So, rather than thinking arrogantly that I could improve the lives and souls of others, I decided to focus more on my own life. I figured that I would then be better equipped for dealing with human situations faced by a physician in patient encounters.

In addition, I have found medical school to be profoundly humbling. I certainly understand now in a way that I never did before how people are able to change very little, either in their own lives or in the lives of others. In some sense I think activism is futile. It isn't just that there will always be more to do — it's that most projects are Band-Aid treatments and simply provide an opportunity to feel good about oneself that isn't justified. . . . Furthermore, I've become numb. So much of what I do as a student is stuff that I don't fully believe in. And rather than try to change everything that I consider wrong in the hospital or the community at large, I just try to get through school in the hope that I will move on to bigger and better things when I have more control over my circumstances. On the other hand, I do believe that habits formed now will rarely be overcome in the future. So I regret not having spoken up on more issues. But I was often too tired.

Andrea wrote that she started out with a "commitment to the well-being of others." This commitment was manifest in her premedical school life. Anyone who interviews medical school applicants can recognize in her words the same motivations expressed by so many others — compassion, sensitivity to the needs of others, a willingness to put oneself on the line, and a sense of optimism about the human condition. However, Andrea (like so many others) found medical school to be "an utter drain." In just a few sentences, she described some of the ways in which she was profoundly changed by her first four years of medical education. Andrea found herself adopting new values, developing a narrower view of life. While she did not entirely abandon her social commitment, Andrea viewed this goal in a more limited and fatalistic fashion. In fact, she concluded that the only way she could achieve anything approximating her original goal was to focus first on helping herself.

We chose to begin this chapter with Andrea's story because it illustrates so well a process that we see happening to most students during the course of their medical education. In this chapter we want to reflect on that story, using our (combined) fifty-plus years as medical educators. In so doing, we will address two sets of questions. The first of these has to do with physicians and individual patients. It includes questions like the following: Why are contemporary physicians seen as dispassionate, distant, or lacking empathy? Why don't they communicate more effectively with their patients? Why are patients frequently dissatisfied with their interactions with physicians? Many people believe that today's doctors just don't "doctor" as well, even though they have considerably more powerful methods of diagnosis and treatment at their disposal.

The second set of questions we will address has to do with community involvement and social activism. This includes questions like the following: Why aren't physicians more involved in health-related community organizations? Why don't more physicians devote themselves professionally to community service? Why aren't physicians more concerned about the inequities of our health care system? These questions are more directly related to the major theme of this book, the relationship between medical education and social consciousness. We believe that there is an important (although by no means necessary) relationship between good doctoring and enhanced social consciousness. Our experience has convinced us that physicians with a high level of altruism and compassion in patient care are more likely to become socially active in the interests of their patients than are those with a low level of these virtues. We suggest that contemporary medical education tends to suppress rather than to foster traditional medical virtues and, in so doing, also tends to suppress social consciousness.

Before we turn to these points, however, an initial point must be made. Even if we are correct that most medical school graduates have an attenuated sense of social commitment, our contention that medical training itself makes them so may be false. The most likely alternative explanation is that the admission process selects applicants with atrophied social dedication. Many critiques of medical education place a great deal of emphasis on the negative aspects of the medical school selection process. They argue that the premedical treadmill gives precedence to science majors with high grades and test scores, who demonstrate personality characteristics like detachment and competitiveness. At the same time the admissions process undervalues the qualitative or affective aspects of the applicants' character or accomplishments. The applicant pool, on this account, is skewed toward individuals who might turn into good scientists or technicians, but who already have two strikes against them when it comes to being compassionate physicians.

Our reason for starting with Andrea's tale is because we believe it is typical. We are convinced that a great majority of the students who matriculate in medical school do, in fact, have the potential to become "good" (i.e., virtuous) doctors. Their self-reported altruism and compassion are usually genuine, although often not mature. Consequently, the "wrong pool of students" explanation for poor outcomes largely misses the boat. Yes, we should try to improve the selection process, but the real problem in medical education lies elsewhere. The situation is reminiscent of the New Testament parable about the farmer who sows good seeds on barren ground. Healthy green shoots arise quickly, but in the absence of nourishment they soon wither. We believe that our entering medical students are good seeds. In this chapter we want to focus on the lack of nourishment and exposure to defoliants they encounter in medical training. How does professional socialization alter the trainee's beliefs and value system so that a "commitment to the well-being of others" either withers or turns into something barely recognizable?

In the next section we briefly discuss the conventional concept of medical virtue, that is, what it has traditionally meant to be a "good physician." In the second section, we show that traditional professional values occupy somewhat the same status in today's medicine as "traditional family values" occupy in American political language. They are honored more in rhetoric than in reality. This leads to a conflict between explicit and tacit teaching about what kind of person a doctor ought to be, and the deleterious consequences of that conflict. The next section focuses on how certain changes already accomplished in medical school admissions policies and curricula may help protect medicine's traditional values and social involvement, at least among some students. The chapter's last section examines the changes taking place in medical training — the

Jack Coulehan and Peter C. Williams

generalist initiative, managed care, ambulatory training — and suggests that some of them may have a favorable influence on tomorrow's medical students and house officers.

Traditional Medical Virtue

Is there a role for social activism in the traditional concept of doctoring? It is important here to distinguish two quite different ways in which social consciousness might be part of the medical persona. In the first, the doctor might draw her professional identity as a healer from commitment to and work for the community as a whole. Here we find public health physicians, physician epidemiologists, or, ironically, the title character in Ibsen's *Enemy of the People*. Andrea might have decided on doctoring because of her desire to maximize the health and welfare of society. In this model her obligations to individual patients would flow from, and perhaps be restricted by, considerations of general welfare. In addition to providing free medical care, many American physicians of the early to mid twentieth century promoted and participated in a wide array of public health activities. For example, community physicians played a major role in the mass polio-immunization campaigns of the early 1950s. Finally, physicians in small towns and rural areas often functioned as civic leaders whose influence was felt in education, welfare, and other nonmedical arenas.

Frankly, very few medical school applicants have this orientation, which is probably just as well for them, since admissions committees actively seek evidence that applicants respond with compassion to the plight of *individual* patients. If applicants' volunteer or work experience has been restricted to education or social welfare, committee members ask, "But how will they respond when confronted with sick people?"

The second way social consciousness has been incorporated into traditional medicine is as a derivative and secondary value. Historically, medical care has focused on the suffering of individual identifiable persons, rather than the overall improvement of health in the community. Yet even though a physician's primary responsibility is to a series of individual patients, meeting this responsibility often requires attention to the social environment from which the patient comes and to which he or she returns. In this sense *some* attention to social context has always been derivatively necessary. Moreover, while historically the good physician has directly demonstrated some social responsibility, the wider concern has been of secondary importance. There was a tradition that physicians would spend some portion of their professional life caring for patients who were unable to pay for their services. This might be a weekly clinic in the local hospital, or it might entail writing off the charges of certain office patients. A late manifestation of pro bono medical care was the "free clinic" movement of the 1960s and 1970s, staffed primarily by volunteer physicians. The ascendancy of Medicare and Medicaid, along with the ethos of specialization, dealt a serious blow to this sense of professional obligation. However, the tradition is still manifest in the AMA Code (9.065), which specifies, "Each physician has an obligation to share in providing care to the indigent. . . . All physicians should work to ensure that the needs of the poor in their communities are met. . . . Caring for the poor should be a regular part of the physician's practice schedule" (AMA, 1996, p. 147). A proportion of physicians carry out these obligations informally in their practices, but the widespread expectation of doing so is long gone.

Moreover, those writing about good doctoring reflect the secondary, albeit real, importance of social consciousness. In *The Virtues in Medical Practice*, Pellegrino and Thomasma (1993) list fidelity, compassion, phronesis, fortitude, temperance, integrity, self-effacement, and justice as primary virtues in medicine. Of nearly one hundred pages on the analysis and implications of these virtues, the authors devote only ten to social justice. Likewise, in *Becoming a Good Doctor: The Place of Virtue and Character in Medical Ethics*, Drane (1988) apportions one out of thirteen chapters to the social aspects of the doctor-patient relationship and access to medical care. This relative weighting is not surprising. Most philosophers of medicine develop their conception of the ends of medicine entirely from what they see as the primary building block of the healing relationship — the individual doctor-patient interaction.

Professional development of medical students during the early to mid part of the twentieth century was generally consistent with this traditional view of medical virtue, including its less important social component. Young men tended to enter the profession with a set of ideals and expectations which, on the whole, were reinforced by the process of professional development. Two aspects of today's medical training — the Flexnerian curriculum, with its division between basic science years and clinical years, and the hierarchical, authoritarian environment — were already well established at that time. Other components of contemporary medical education were yet to develop — in particular, the full-time physician-scientist as a primary role model, the remarkable dependence on distance-producing technology, and the extraordinary bureaucratization of care. The synergism between professional values and educational environment was marked by the *presence* of certain professional expectations which are less common today (e.g., self-sacrifice, long hours of work, difficult working conditions, social regard and utility), as well as the *absence* of other expectations (e.g., ex-

Jack Coulehan and Peter C. Williams

aggerated social power, extremely high income), which have become common today.

We believe that a major change took place from the 1950s through 1970s as a result of the changing medical school environment and social expectations. As a result of these changes, contemporary medical training is less likely to foster social consciousness in either of its forms (primary or secondary), and professional socialization is also less likely to nourish the basic attributes of "good" doctoring.

Professional Development Today

The structure and process of contemporary medical education are well known. Initially, students study medically related sciences taught by research scientists rather than physicians. Acquisition of information is the dominant thrust. After demonstrating an ability to recount immense amounts of data, students begin what is essentially an apprenticeship — more often run by more advanced apprentices than masters. In recent decades this ninety-year-old Flexnerian curriculum has been modified in two major ways. First, many medical schools have adopted programs or curricula that allow students to have some clinical exposure during the basic science years. This generally amounts to courses in medical interviewing and clinical examination but sometimes also includes continuity experiences in a clinic or preceptor's office. Second, some medical schools have adopted aspects of new curricula based on principles of adult learning. This approach, pioneered in the 1970s by McMaster University's problem-based learning (PBL) curriculum, became politically feasible when Harvard adopted its New Pathway in the mid 1980s. In its purest form, the PBL venue abandons lectures, examinations, and other traditional teacher-driven techniques and relies solely on a small-group tutorial approach in which students assume the responsibility of "working through" a simulated clinical case. With Harvard's success widely touted, many medical schools have adopted some components or variations of PBL into their preclinical curricula. PBL is said to enhance the educational process because the learning (i.e., derived from clinical cases) and skills (i.e., in some sense approximating clinical decision making) are more relevant. These claims are controversial. Even if true, however, PBL in itself does not significantly alter the features of medical education with which we are most concerned in this chapter.

In the hospital, the major role models for students are residents or, worse, attending physicians whose primary commitment is to subspecialty practice and clinical research, rather than to the day-to-day care of patients. In both preclinical and clinical spheres, there has been a very strong emphasis on scientific knowledge as the "Rosetta stone" for understanding other forms of human discourse. In this context medical language largely replaces other forms of communication. The emotional (affective) aspects of human experience are distanced and diminished. Technical skills are considered fundamental, while interactive skills (if encouraged at all) are secondary. The dominant style of teaching is authoritative, hence hierarchical and authoritarian. The power structure implicitly, and often explicitly, devalues primary medical care and relationship-centered approaches to practicing medicine. This takes place in a hothouse atmosphere which is often psychologically and spiritually brutal, as indicated in Andrea's statement: "The people are rude, the hours are long, there is a test at the end of virtually every rotation." Trainee abuse includes long work hours and intense, conflicting demands, associated with a general lack of emotional support from faculty and role model physicians.

Much has been written about professional socialization in this environment (Bloom, 1989; Hafferty & Franks, 1994; Hundert, 1996; Manson, 1994; Petersdorf, 1992; Wear, 1997). As students and house officers successfully wend their way through often negative experiences, they gradually adopt the professional culture and its value system as their own. An important aspect of this socialization is the transfer of a set of beliefs and values regarding what it means to be a good physician. This learning process includes both tacit and explicit components. What we call *tacit learning* includes all those aspects of the curriculum and the socialization process that instill professional values and a sense of professional identity, but do so without explicitly talking about those issues. Thus, tacit learning arises from what Hafferty and Franks call the "hidden curriculum" (1994) in medical training or from Hundert's "informal curriculum" (1996). The former concept is more inclusive, however, because "it includes the hidden transmission of the dominant culture during formal classes, whereas the informal curriculum is that subset of the hidden curriculum that happens outside classes, hospital rounds and the like" (Hafferty & Franks, 1994, p. 861).

Alternatively, the *explicit learning* component of professional development includes courses, classes, discussion on rounds, advice, or other teaching that is overtly intended to instill professional values. Beginning in the 1970s most medical schools introduced biomedical ethics into their formal curriculum. Ethics courses frequently address issues of professional identity and medical virtue. Humanities courses typically articulate the virtues or attributes associated with being a "good" physician and the special moral obligations that arise in the physician-patient relationship. In addition, some of these courses consider social

Jack Coulehan and Peter C. Williams

issues in medicine and the role of physicians in society. In many medical schools nonphysicians teach courses in medical ethics and humanities. Additional explicit learning occurs in the clinical setting, where attending physicians offer more informal but no less direct cautionary statements about how to behave in medical practice. Ideally, these explicit elements of the curriculum would be consistent with the tacit learning that occurs throughout medical training. However, all the evidence to date indicates that they are not.

The tacit socialization process goes on continuously, day after day, throughout medical training. Tacit learning is much more powerful than explicit learning not only because it is reinforced more frequently but because it relates to *doing* rather than *saying*. As an example of this process, consider basic notions of how compassion manifests itself in the care of patients. The explicit curriculum stresses the development of empathy and associated listening and responding skills, the relief of suffering, the importance of trust and fidelity, and a primary focus on the patient's best interest. Tacit learning, on the other hand, stresses objectivity, detachment, wariness, and distrust of emotions, patients, payors, hospital administration, and the state. In their clinical education students become cynical about the value of tenderness and virtue because they learn that they can better survive the slings and arrows of clinical training by developing an "us versus them" mentality where almost everyone else is "them." Worst of all, patients are potential enemies, or at least inconvenient objects instead of suffering subjects. Andrea Fricchione, who began her education with a high level of personal and social concern, concluded after years of tacit socialization that her own needs must come first since activism is "futile" and she had to conserve her energy to deal with patient interactions. This conflict between tacit and explicit values distorts medical professionalism.

In particular, tacit learning favors the development of three characteristics or traits that make it difficult to be a caring physician. The first is *detachment*. The notion that detachment is a prime requisite for objectivity in medicine is questionable (Coulehan, 1996, 1997). Good medical practice can better be characterized as a tension between engagement and detachment. The constant emphasis on detachment encourages physicians to discount the affective and imaginative aspects of their work, while focusing exclusively on the cognitive and technical aspects. Because so much of one's self is invested in the professional milieu (especially during training), one's affective skills may atrophy, resulting in a state of emotional numbness. In the first chapter of his *Medical Ethics*, Thomas Percival enjoins physicians to "unite tenderness with steadiness" in their care of patients (in Leake, 1927). By the term "steadiness" we interpret Percival to mean the intellectual virtue of objectivity or reason, along with the moral virtue of courage or fortitude. By the term "tenderness" we interpret him to mean humanity, compassion, empathy, and sympathy. Elsewhere Percival contrasts the "coldness of heart" that often develops in practitioners who do not cultivate such virtues with the "tender charity" that the moral practice of medicine requires (in Baker, 1993). We believe that the emphasis on detachment in medical training promotes such "coldness of heart." When coupled with the structure of clinical training — overwork, shift work, ineffective or "unaffective" mentoring — the tendency to withdraw is overwhelming.

The second characteristic is a strong sense of *entitlement*. Physicians-in-training have every right to believe that the social utility of their work demands respect. However, the duration, rigor, intensity, and abusiveness of today's medical education also engender a sense of entitlement to high income, prestige, and social power. In essence, medical trainees believe that physicians have to pay very high "dues" — tuition, long hours, deferred gratification, great responsibility — which then warrants their receiving very high benefits in return. This set of beliefs is usually superimposed on an underlying humanitarian ethic. In most cases, altruism, compassion, and desire to help others played a large part in the trainees' choice of profession and continues, both consciously and unconsciously, to play a role in self-image. Nonetheless, the belief that "I do this to serve others" often coexists with, and obscures, the belief that "I *deserve* high rewards for my work."

During the 1970s and 1980s the sense of entitlement was strongly reinforced by reality. Physicians had great power, not only by virtue of rapid progress in medical science (Aesculapian power, to use Howard Brody's term [1992]), but also because society seemed to grant progressively greater cultural significance to medicine (social power). In a society dedicated to cheating death, physicians were cultural icons — great warriors, intrepid heroes, and wise counselors. As we will discuss below, the development of managed care has diminished certain aspects of medical power (e.g., income level and autonomy), and in the 1990s cultural images of physician have turned increasingly sour (e.g., doctors are insensitive clods or money-grubbing providers). No wonder physicians with a strong sense of entitlement grounded in the 1970s and 1980s have reacted so negatively to these changes. We believe the outrage may be fueled as much (or more) by injured entitlement as it is by legitimate concern for patients in the managed care environment.

In addition to detachment and entitlement, the third characteristic fostered by contemporary medical education is a phenomenon we call *nonreflective professionalism*. This is a belief system by which physicians can consciously adhere to traditional medical values, while at the same time adopting beliefs and practices at variance with these values. It is the gap between professional values the doctor believes he or she holds and professional values manifest in his or her behavior. To describe what we mean by this term, it is helpful to survey the different ways in which medical trainees might reconcile the conflicting messages of tacit and explicit learning. We identify three broad categories of response: deflation of values, conflation of values, and maintenance of values.

The first approach is for trainees to adapt their conception of the ideal physician to fit their actual experience and the socialization process responsible for it. In other words, they discard traditional medical virtues. They become cynical about concepts like duty, fidelity, confidentiality, and integrity. They question their own motivations and those of their patients. These physicians take on an "objective" professional identity that generally narrows their sphere of responsibility and confines it to the technical arena. Given this ethos, statements like the following make perfect sense: "He's an extremely good doctor, but he sure is nasty with patients." "Her bedside manner is terrible, but she's the best gastroenterologist in the city." To those who subscribe to this ethic, being a "good" doctor is a technical accomplishment that cannot be compromised by lack of sensitivity, communication skills, or any professional virtue other than competence.

A second, and we believe considerably more frequent, method of resolving the discrepancy between tacit and explicit learning is to adopt a nonreflective professional identity or nonreflective professionalism, in which one holds that behaviors deriving from the tacit set of values are, in fact, the best way to manifest the explicit values. Thus, young medical professionals become convinced that the most effective way to show compassion for a patient is to take a clinically detached approach. Likewise, the nonreflective professional identity tends to conflate self-interest with the patient's interest. Physicians convince themselves that behaviors favored in the hospital's culture of survival best serve the interests of their patients in the long run. In general, this involves substituting technological intervention for personal interaction. Because culturally we associate benefit with "providing the best" and "being aggressive," patients usually expect (or at least accept) their physicians' predilection toward performing too many, rather than too few, interventions. It requires considerably less personal involvement for a physician to do *something* (for example, prescribe an antibiotic or order an x-ray) in a situation where simple advice or continued observation might be the better approach. Until the recent managed care revolution, this pattern of aggressive diagnosis and treatment also resulted in economic and social benefits for the physician. In other words, nonreflective physicians could view themselves as championing patient benefit while at the same time pursuing doctor-benefit practices.

Andrea Fricchione's statement demonstrates some of these characteristics. First, she says she became convinced that giving of herself to improve the lives of others was a type of "arrogance." This arrogance was defused by the "profoundly humbling" experience of medical school, which conveyed the (tacit) message that "people can't change so you're wasting your time." (We found this remark of Andrea's particularly ironic, since it spoke of a profound change in *her* during her tenure at our school.) In this situation, how could she best achieve her original goal? The only solution was to focus on her own needs ("hoarding my extra time for simple pleasures"). This strategy would leave her "better equipped" for the frustrations she faced — presumably the best result in a bad situation. Andrea hadn't abandoned her explicit values ("the best thing I could do for my patients, for my fellow human being . . ."), but she had decided that by decreasing her personal involvement with them, or her professional commitments in general, she would actually benefit them more.

A third group of medical trainees escapes or avoids succumbing to the conflict between tacit and explicit socialization. In some sense they seem to be "immunized" against the forces that undermine medical virtue. These students progress through medical school and postgraduate training while not only maintaining but also often nourishing an altruistic professional persona. In this case the seed either falls on a patch of good soil, or is a superhybrid seed that thrives on adversity. What factors might help students resist becoming narrow or nonreflective physicians? Some seem to have natural immunity; others benefit from immunization.

In our experience a strong predictor of natural immunization is the student's commitment to a set of standards or principles beyond the ideals of medicine. Such commitment tends to protect the student from the negative values instilled by tacit socialization into the practice of medicine. For example, students who identify strongly with their religious tradition, and practice it, may more easily stave off detachment and fragmentation in their professional lives. The trend toward admitting a greater number of "nontraditional" applicants to medical school may have increased the pool of students committed to higher ideals. Nontraditional applicants include those with humanities, rather than science, degrees. Though the connection is surely contingent, training in the humanities, unlike the more quantitative disciplines, demands a kind of self-reflection and self-expression that, in our mind, fosters altruism. Another class of non-

Jack Coulehan and Peter C. Williams

traditional student that seems less prone to nonreflective professionalism is the older student, who has had additional life experience, either in different careers or in postcollege projects (e.g., Peace Corps, teaching in low-income-area schools, and public policy fellowships). Andrea fit into both categories. Such students may have already tested their altruism and caring in other endeavors. In some cases their postcollege work may have required the courage to drop out of the mainstream to achieve a personal objective. In other cases the switch to medicine may have required the courage to give up promising and lucrative jobs. Presumably such nontraditional students bring a more defined and mature mixture of values to the medical school mix.

Three additional trends in medical schools over the last twenty years might prima facie have resulted in a higher percentage of students being "naturally" resistant to dehumanizing forces. The first was the greatly increasing percentage of female students. Since women are socialized from childhood to be more empathic and compassionate, they presumably enter medical training with a greater reservoir of caring skills and more openness to learning the affective and interpersonal aspects of doctoring. There is now considerable evidence that at least in the primary care specialties women physicians tend to spend more time with and communicate more effectively with their patients than do their male peers.

The second trend is the family medicine movement, which really got off the ground in the early to mid 1970s and by the 1990s had extended (to a greater or lesser extent) to almost all of the U.S. medical schools. While traditional specialties viewed family medicine in terms of its *depth* (i.e., less knowledge in a given area), family medicine promoted itself on the basis of *breadth* (i.e., its wide range of subject matter). Moreover, family medicine argued that the whole is greater than the sum of its parts; caring for the whole person requires more than a certain level of knowledge and skill in various disease-oriented specialties.

The movement seized upon George Engel's biopsychosocial model to describe its philosophy. In a classic 1977 *Science* article, Engel characterized modern medicine as based on a reductionistic model; that is, it focused on reducing the human organism to its component biological parts. As an alternative, he proposed a general systems theory approach that was grounded in the complex interaction among various organizational levels, both "below" (biological) and "above" (social, cultural) the whole person. The heuristic that Engels coined (i.e., biopsychosocial) rapidly caught on among medical educators who were promoting family medicine or primary care, as well as those interested in community medicine and public health. In particular, family medicine departments added behavioral scientists to their faculties, and communication skills, psychosocial medicine, and a variety of other humanistic components to their curricula. In family medicine the explicit values of caring for the whole person-as-person were synergistic with the tacit values inculcated by the training culture.

The third potentially beneficial trend was the establishment of medical humanities teaching in the majority of medical schools. Knight (1995) identified two of these factors — the greater number of female students and the introduction of medical humanities courses — as positive influences in the moral environment of medical education in recent decades. However, in their commentary on Knight's paper, Brody, Squier, and Foglio (1995) questioned this conclusion, at least as far as medical humanities are concerned. They argue (as we do) that the medical ethics and humanities movement has not necessarily made medical education more humane, although it certainly has provided some useful resources for doing so.

There are several limitations to medical ethics and humanities courses as "immunizers" against nonreflective professionalism. The first limitation is quantitative. Ethics courses are often relatively short and taught in the preclinical rather than clinical curriculum. The student may learn useful information about such topics as advance directives, informed consent, surrogate decision making, and confidentiality, but this constitutes only an initial dose that may not be reinforced (or may be suppressed by conflicting information) when the student enters his or her clinical life. A second limitation is qualitative. While end-of-life decision making and other areas of quandary ethics are important topics, professional values inform every aspect of day-to-day medical practice. Empathy, compassion, attentiveness, fidelity, courage — these values are not easily communicated by "hard" ethics courses, no matter how intensive or well placed. By the same token, these virtues are hard to develop "on the run" in a clinical factory in which time for reflection, interaction, and feedback are scarce. If they can be learned in coursework at all, they may more likely be nourished in "softer" humanities courses such as literature, film, or religious studies, where analysis, reflection, and self-awareness are central. Whatever else is said, the skills involved (i.e., listening, empathic responding) must be explicitly taught in courses on interviewing and physician-patient communication.

The third, and most important, limitation combines quantitative and qualitative features. As we have argued, the culture of clinical training is relatively hostile to professional virtue. Because the tacit value system of the hospital is so potent in forming the trainee's view of doctoring, the explicit values embodied in ethics and humanities courses may have little impact (Erde, 1997). For example, in her medical ethics course a student may have learned a great deal about informed consent — its four components, the relevant ethical and legal arguments, and the judicial standards by which consent is judged. Furthermore, in her course on physician-patient communication, the same student may have learned the appropriate methods of facilitating or negotiating informed consent. These topics are in the explicit curriculum. However, in her surgical clerkship she may encounter a culture in which none of this material is particularly relevant. The surgical residents may think that consent is a mere formality. Her attending surgeon may boast that informed consent is a farce, and he can get a patient to agree to anything he wants: "It's not what you say, it's how you say it." Moreover, the pace and pressure of work are such that there is no time to spend educating patients or answering their questions. The tacit value system embedded in this culture is far different from and often contrary to the explicit value system the student learned — but it's the system in which she is immersed during the most crucial months (and, later, years) of her transformation into a physician.

Thus, the third limitation is that ethics and humanities curricula are largely irrelevant unless they have a substantive and continuing impact on hospital culture. Frequent ethics rounds and ethics conferences on clinical services are a step in the right direction, but if run primarily by "ethics specialists," these may have little impact. The idea, of course, is to infiltrate the culture by coopting residents and attendings — first obtaining their goodwill, then fanning goodwill into enthusiasm. If an ethics program can somehow achieve a critical mass of "values sensitive" clinical faculty, it may begin to influence the institution's ethos.

The Medicine in Contemporary Society (MCS) curriculum at Stony Brook has had some — albeit limited — success accomplishing this at our University Hospital and Medical Center (Coulehan, Williams, & Naser, 1995; Coulehan, Williams, Landis, & Naser, 1995). First, MCS is an extensive program that includes fifty-six-hour required courses in each of the first two years of medical school; exercises in several of the third-year clerkships; and a required project or course during the fourth year. The sheer quantity of time devoted to MCS signals its institutional importance. Second, the courses integrate topics, materials, and techniques from a variety of disciplines — history, literature, film, and sociology — rather than focusing solely on ethics and law. Third, our courses are primarily small-group experiences in which nine or ten students interact with two faculty members, at least one of whom is a practicing physician. With ten groups in the first-year course and ten in the second, we recruit approximately forty volunteer faculty each year to serve as facilitators. These include physicians from diverse specialties — anesthesiology, dermatology, family medicine, surgery, internal medicine, radiology, and pathology. Our regular faculty meetings and annual retreats constitute a faculty development program, and help build a relatively large pool of clinicians whose preclinical teaching may help transform (if, in fact, it needs to be transformed) their teaching and practice in the hospital and clinic. To return to a distinction we drew earlier, though the manifest purpose of MCS is to train students, our own "hidden curriculum" in this course is to train the cadre of *faculty* necessary for any program in professionalism to succeed in an institutional setting.

What are the results of the MCS humanities immersion? (It's actually just a dip, but compared to the standard medical curriculum, it is an immersion and, for some students, close to a drowning.) We have to admit there is no "hard" evidence that Stony Brook graduates are more likely to practice traditional medical virtues or to be more socially involved than medical graduates are in general. Our rate of incarcerated graduates is about at the national norm. Our school remains about average in the percentage of graduates who choose primary care specialties, though, interestingly, it has a remarkably high number of graduates who choose careers in academic medicine. Our graduates do tend to have good background knowledge of medical ethics, health law, and communication skills. Because students invest so much time and energy in MCS, the course has become an identifiable part of student culture at Stony Brook. At times MCS remains the butt of jokes, a target of anger, or an object of disdain for some students, but most students enthusiastically endorse it. In the preclinical years, MCS sometimes provides an oasis of care and reflectiveness in an otherwise hostile environment. The courses and requirements have sufficient weight that they cannot be "blown off" or, at least, students have to work hard to dismiss them. On the whole, we believe the MCS program has been visible and persuasive enough that it has been able to influence Stony Brook's clinical culture.

Don't forget, however, that resistance to detachment, entitlement, and nonreflective professionalism is relative — while it may affect many students, perhaps only a few of them become completely immune. Andrea Fricchione had several "doses" — she is a woman, she had a nontraditional background, she (originally, at least) intended to go into family medicine, and she not only completed our MCS curriculum, she was an enthusiastic participant. Nonetheless, she succumbed to a diagnosable case of nonreflective professionalism.

Where Do We Go from Here?

Medical education stands at the doorstep of profound change. Academic medical centers are already being forced to step through that door into an uncertain and potentially hostile new environment. These changes have nothing to do with scholarly analysis or self-reflection, but rather are a direct consequence of the revolution in health care financing for which we use the general term "managed care." Among the most important features of the new system is a corporate mentality in which much of the "fat" of traditional medical education must be eliminated. Specifically, clinical faculty will have to spend more time practicing medicine more efficiently, and less time performing nonreimbursable tasks, such as teaching, scholarship, or nonfunded research. Moreover, organizational changes in the new health care system will favor primary care education at the expense of residency and fellowship positions in subspecialty areas and clinical training in ambulatory settings rather than the hospital.

Some commentators claim that the corporate transformation of medical care may lead to the decline and death of traditional professional values, such as fidelity, altruism, confidentiality, and integrity (Kassirer, 1998). The concern that self-interest will be encouraged in "mercantilized" medicine has a priori plausibility. Likewise, physicians' social commitments, whether to the social dimension of patient welfare or to the community as a whole, may wither as physicians progressively adopt a business mentality (Zoloth-Dorfman & Rubin, 1995). Since we have argued that, for the last thirty years or more, the powerful tacit socialization process in medical education has *already* damaged doctoring, we can retain some optimism that the managed care revolution can't make it much worse. Granted, the 1980s subspecialist was trained as an *impresario* technician, rather than an *employee* technician, but he or she already lived in an environment in which traditional values tended to be suppressed, rather than enhanced. Most physicians, to some extent at least, held a nonreflective view of professionalism. Thus, the notion that managed care will diminish a presumably high level of medical virtue seems naive. To the contrary, managed care may gouge the heart out of certain medical vices, such as arrogance and sense of entitlement. Nonetheless, there is little question that managed care has important ethical implications (AMA, 1995; Holleman, Holleman, & Moy, 1997; Miles & Koepp, 1995).

What are the likely effects of the corporate transformation of medicine on medical curricula? It seems probable that the new emphasis on primary care will lead to more training in the knowledge, skills, and values associated with day-to-day interaction with patients. More of the clinical curriculum will take place in the ambulatory setting. More of it may be taught by nonclinicians who will be comparatively more available for teaching. There will probably be fewer residency and fellowship positions in certain surgical and procedure-oriented subspecialties. In medical school the curricula will include more attention to outcomes studies, evidence-based medicine, quality assessment, clinical guidelines, and health care economics. Combined degree programs (e.g., M.D.-M.B.A. and

M.D.-M.P.H.) might become more common to meet the growing need for physician administrators.

With regard to the explicit professional values curriculum, it seems unlikely that *less* attention will be paid to medical ethics, humanities, and social issues in medicine. Lectures, seminars, conferences, and courses supporting medical and social values will probably accompany the trends outlined in the preceding paragraph. Managed care has, if anything, made the social *interdependence* of medicine more explicit. Physicians will come to see themselves and their patients in the context of a multiplicity of social values and institutions, rather than as isolated players. Thus, the type of curriculum exemplified by Stony Brook's Medicine in Contemporary Society courses would seem to be at least as relevant, if not more relevant, than in the past. From this perspective, it seems at least plausible that future physicians of the twenty-first century will be more socially aware than today's physicians are because they will be socialized to be more *connected*.

If we accept these general considerations as valid, what additional changes in medical education might realistically promote increased social consciousness and activism among physicians? We suggest the following:

Admissions policy. To a large extent the social context of medical practice determines the expectations of those who choose to enter the profession. For example, those who studied medicine in the 1970s and 1980s believed that physicians were entitled to substantial independence and high income. Those who elect to study medicine in the managed care era will approach it with a different set of expectations. It is quite possible that the number of applicants will decrease and, from the standpoint of traditional indices like MCAT scores, the pool will become less competitive.

Two features of the medical school application process are of special note. First, admissions committees expect students to express in their extracurricular activities a concern for the well-being of the community of patients. As we noted earlier, application essays often describe both a commitment to and experience with social activism. Recent essays reviewed by the authors are typical in indicating awareness of "the role economics plays in health and access to health care," "social as well as physical health," "the role social context plays in care giving." Moreover, virtually all applicants hope to demonstrate their altruism by volunteering their time and efforts — at crisis hotlines, emergency rooms, ambulance corps, tutoring programs. Surely sophisticated students realize that admission committees are responsive to statements and activities like these, but unless one considers these applicants hypocritical, we want to reiterate that most students enter medical school with a genuine concern for the community of patients. We argued earlier that the implicit socialization process tends to sup-

Jack Coulehan and Peter C. Williams

press these values. In the future applicants may be even more committed to medical virtue because other expectations will be lower. When they enter medical school, these students may well encounter a socialization process more supportive of, or at least not so hostile to, altruism, compassion, and social awareness.

Secondly, if medicine becomes less lucrative with fewer opportunities for independence and power, men may be less drawn to the field. If the rather speculative correlation we have drawn between gender and loss of social concern is correct, the increasing percentage of women in the field bodes well for American health care.

Preclinical curriculum. The preclinical curriculum in American medical schools has become a pressure cooker — too much information, too little time, too many attempts to repackage, and too few clear educational goals. We believe that the trends toward integration of material across disciplines — both internal to medicine and across professions — and problem-based learning will continue, although pure examples will probably not be adopted by most medical schools both for practical reasons and educational considerations. In this time of decreasing faculty resources, problem-based learning may not be feasible in many schools. Moreover, its educational advantages as a complete system are at present unclear. The basic principles — for example, active learning in small groups — are, however, well established.

Irrespective of how the basic sciences are taught, the preclinical curriculum should include a substantive multidisciplinary track that deals with social issues in medicine. This offering ought to include the physician-patient relationship, traditional virtues of physicians, socialization in medical education, literature and medicine, medical ethics, health law, anthropology, ethnomedicine, and health economics, especially the structure and function of the health care delivery system.

The preclinical curriculum should also be redesigned to include socially relevant *doing* as well as *studying*. The current opportunities for "clinical exposure" during the first and second year in most medical schools do not satisfy this requirement. From the students' perspective, of course, interacting with patients in the hospital or office setting is highly desirable, but does not necessarily supplement the tacit learning environment to include concepts of interdisciplinary practice, biopsychosocial modeling, and social responsibility. The AMA Code of Medical Ethics (in section 7) specifies that "a physician shall recognize a responsibility to participate in activities contributing to an improved community." In another section (3) it indicates that "a physician shall . . . recognize a responsibility to seek changes in (legal) requirements which are contrary to the best interests of the patient." If these requirements are important manifestations of professionalism, they should be addressed in medical education. In our model, students would select from a menu of available programs, choosing experiences that fit with their own interests and skills. These might include, for example, HIV education in local high schools, volunteer work in hospices, health services for migrant farm workers, or even work with environmental or other politically active volunteer organizations.

Clinical training. The clinical curriculum at many medical schools has already been expanded to give students experience in a broader array of clinical settings. Stony Brook, like many medical schools, now requires that students spend time in both the third and fourth years working in primary care, and also that the traditional third-year clerkships provide more of their teaching in outpatient settings. In addition to these broad requirements, curricula will need to address neglected topic areas that will enhance the relevance of clinical training to contemporary practice. Since most patients will soon be cared for under managed care contracts, it makes sense that the objectives, organization, and function of managed care be added to clinical training. In fact, health care assessment, quality assurance, and peer review — topics traditionally absent from medical training — should now be taught in concert with other aspects of the contemporary "management" of medical services. Evidence-based medicine is another set of knowledge and skills that should be integrated into the clinical curriculum.

The self-contained blocks of clinical training are necessary for organization and efficiency, but there is no reason that students might not have longitudinal commitments along with their rotations and block electives. One such commitment would certainly be the opportunity to develop long-term relationships with primary care patients and chronically ill or disabled patients. Likewise, there should be an expectation that students continue their preclinical work with the same (or a different) social welfare agency or other community activity. An evaluation by their "social preceptor" should be included as part of their clinical portfolio along with clerkship grades and evaluations.

We want to make it clear once again that U.S. physicians emerge from their medical training with a wide array of professional beliefs and values. Many physicians are thoughtful and introspective. Many are exemplary in their devotion to patient welfare — individual and collective. Some bring to their work a broad view of social responsibility. Nonetheless, we contend that U.S. medical education in recent decades has favored 1) a conscious commitment to traditional values of doctoring — empathy, compassion, and altruism among them; 2) a tacit commitment to behaviors grounded in an ethic of detachment, self-interest, and objectivity; and 3) an implicit avowal that they best care for their patients by treating them as objects of technical services (medical care). This collection of values impairs doctoring and inhibits social activism.

Medical education is characterized in part by this conflict between explicit and tacit professional values. Some trainees respond by reconceptualizing themselves primarily as technicians and narrowing their professional identity to an ethic of competence. Others develop nonreflective professionalism, as we have illustrated with the story of Andrea Fricchione.

Some features of medical education in the last two decades have tended to immunize trainees against nonreflective professionalism, or to ameliorate it. The trainee's beliefs, gender, background, and character may make a difference. The development of family medicine and the biopsychosocial model has created an alternative culture within mainstream medicine. This serves as an oasis for others. The almost universal adoption of the biomedical ethics movement has also had some influence. However, ethics courses are generally small parts of the explicit curriculum and, as such, have little impact on the tacit aspects of hospital culture. Broader-based humanities curricula, especially if they enlist a large cohort of clinical faculty and are integrated into clinical training, are likely to be more effective.

Changes in the culture of medicine in the last forty years have had their epicenter in medical schools and teaching hospitals, but they also reflect the profession's increased affluence and social power. The locus of change has now shifted to ambulatory settings and the marketplace. It remains to be seen whether this move will lessen the disjunction between the values of the explicit curriculum and the manifestly contradictory ones taught day to day during patient care, among them detachment, entitlement, and a belief that the patient's interest coincides with the physician's interest.

PART TWO

Shaping the Experience of Medical Education

SHEILA WOODS
SUE FOSSON
LOIS MARGARET NORA

Student Advocacy for a Culture of Professionalism at the University of Kentucky College of Medicine

Since its founding, the College of Medicine at the University of Kentucky has emphasized community service as part of the professional ethics of being a physician. Curricular reform in the early 1990s reinforced our focus on professionalism. In 1996, we placed additional emphasis on professionalism in our training environment with our Medical Professionalism Project. This project is an excellent example of the involvement of medical students in shaping a project that, in turn, shapes their environment.

From the graduation of its first class in 1964, the University of Kentucky College of Medicine has shown a commitment to community service as a fundamental professional ethic of physicians. Particularly in rural states, physicians play crucial community service roles. At UK, these roles are fostered through formal training as well as through extracurricular activities.

UK's medical curriculum is interdisciplinary, emphasizing the early acquisition of clinical skills, integration of basic science and clinical disciplines, and active learning techniques. Professionalism is included in learning objectives throughout the curriculum, particularly in the course "Introduction to the Medical Profession" and the two-year-long course "Patients, Physicians, and Society." Using case-based instruction, standardized patients, and resource persons from the community, students encounter a variety of legal, ethical, socioeconomic, and societal issues.

All first-year students complete a clinical preceptorship with a primary care physician. Many of our students comment during debriefing sessions on their surprise at how involved in community service their preceptors are. Particularly in rural counties, physicians serve in multiple service roles, such as school board member, sports team physician, or library board member, in addition to their medical practice. In their clinical training, students spend a minimum of eight weeks in rural sites, and a minimum of twelve weeks in primary care practices. Thus, the exposure to community service as a way of professional life is continually reinforced.

In the integrated Women's Maternal and Child Health Clerkship, students rotate in a weekly pediatric clinic for uninsured patients run by a local mission. Also, as part of this clerkship, students become actively involved in the Young Parents Program, a learning experience that combines social service with key learning objectives in obstetrics, gynecology, and pediatrics. While caring for a pregnant adolescent, all students assist in prenatal care, participate in the delivery of the young mother, and are active in postnatal education, health care delivery sessions, and the baby's well-child visits.

Our informal curriculum reinforces the centrality of community service to professionalism. Since the inception of the school, all medical school classes elect one or more community service representatives in addition to the more traditional class officers of president, vice president, secretary, and treasurer. These class officer(s) are responsible for integrating community service into student life. Each class individually or in cooperation with other classes completes one or more community service projects each year. Projects have included blood drives, Toys for Tots, clothing collections, and Project Read. These class-based community service activities also provide a mechanism for medical students to involve faculty, administrative staff, and others in service projects.

Other examples of medical student involvement in the community abound. A medical clinic based at the Salvation Army has offered opportunities for practitioners and students from a variety of health disciplines to provide needed health care in the Lexington area. Students work as volunteers at the Hope Center, a local homeless shelter. An HIV/AIDS Teaching Project brings volunteer medical students into area schools to provide factual information about HIV and AIDS and instruction about high-risk behaviors. As a part of the Women's Maternal and Child Health Clerkship, all students spend a day in a high school leading small-group discussions with local high school students on risk-taking behaviors in adolescence.

Community service as an aspect of professionalism is also a feature of the Service Learning Interdisciplinary Project at the University of Kentucky. Based in the College of Nursing, the Service Learning Project includes students from medicine, nursing, pharmacy, dentistry, and the allied health professions. Each team of students works with a community organization to help that organization complete an internal needs assessment; the team then responds to one or more of the identified needs. This project also teaches teamwork and respect for the other health care disciplines. Out of this service learning program a number of projects have emerged, including a community health fair, dental examinations brought into local schools, a playground designed and built at a shelter for abused mothers and children, and a "brown bag" day at a local mission clinic where patients brought in their medications for explanations about possible interactions. This latter program, organized by pharmacy students and medical students, proved such a success that it is now a routine service provided for patients of this mission clinic.

Despite the successes of these various programs, in 1996 the school determined that professionalism demanded more focused attention. This recognition began with a reconsideration of our honor code policy, which highlighted the need for peer evaluation to begin early in training. Other realizations pertained to the changing economic pressures faced by clinicians and researchers in our environment, awareness of the expanded role played by other health professionals in patient care, and the increasing presence of managed care and associated challenges to the traditional patient-doctor relationship. As the need for more focus on these aspects of professionalism became apparent, the Office of Academic Affairs at the University of Kentucky College of Medicine instituted the Professionalism Project.

––––––––

We began by establishing a Task Force on Professionalism, including medical students, faculty from basic and clinical sciences, and community physicians. The dean appointed fifteen members, based on their interest in humanism and professionalism in medicine. A clinician with special interest in humanism in medicine and the assistant dean of student affairs assumed leadership of the task force. The overall goal was to ensure the integrity of the profession of medicine and the excellent quality of health care provided to patients. In addition, the dean charged the task force to devise a working definition of professionalism in medicine. Drawing on a literature review and the American Board of Internal Medicine's *Project Professionalism* (1995), the task force met three different times to come up with a definition of professionalism upon which everyone — medical students, basic science and clinical faculty, and administration — could agree. The definition is as follows:

> The University of Kentucky College of Medicine regards professionalism and humanism in the training of medical students to be an essential goal. Throughout the curriculum, medical students are exposed to professional behavior issues, moral and ethical decision making, and community service opportunities. The following definition of professionalism is UKCOM's guideline by which professional behavior expectations are set. These expectations apply to all medical students as well as faculty, and begin with matriculation in medical school.

Professionalism includes altruism, accountability, excellence, duty, service, honor and integrity, and respect for others. Definitions of these concepts have been developed by the American Board of Internal Medicine's Project Professionalism and are listed below.

Altruism: Physicians must serve the best interests of patients above their own interests.

Accountability: Physicians are accountable to their patients for fulfilling the implied contract governing the patient-physician relationship. They are also accountable to society for addressing the health needs of the public and to their profession to uphold medicine's ethical precepts.

Excellence: Physicians must make a conscientious effort to exceed ordinary expectations and maintain lifelong learning.

Duty: Physicians must accept a commitment to serve their patients. Accepting inconveniences to meet the needs of one's patients, enduring unavoidable personal risk, advocating for care regardless of ability to pay, and volunteering one's skills and expertise for the welfare of the community are all part of the accepted duty.

Honor and integrity: Honor and integrity imply being fair, being truthful, keeping one's word, meeting commitments, and being straightforward.

Respect for others: Demonstrating respect for patients, their families, other physicians and health care professionals is the essence of humanism. Humanism is essential in the practice of medicine.

Next, the task force completed an environmental needs assessment with data obtained from students, patients, faculty, and administrators. Data from medical students came from three sources. First, we examined our students' responses in comparison to the national mean for the AAMC Graduating Student Questionnaire on rating "how well your clinical faculty demonstrated and exemplified the following skills and attitudes." The results were as follows:

	UK Students	National Mean
Altruism	2.1	2.1
Integrity	1.8	1.8
Compassion	1.9	1.9
Honesty	1.7	1.8
Professionalism	1.7	1.7

(Scale of 1 = excellent to 4 = poor)

We concluded that our faculty performed at the mean in students' estimations.

Second, the class of 1999 completed surveys concerning their experiences in third-year clerkships, the previous academic year. The attitudes of the majority of students changed for the better toward attending faculty and residents. But 46 percent of students reported observing unethical conduct by resident physicians, and 26 percent of students reported observing unethical conduct by attending faculty. Ninety-six percent of students reported hearing derogatory comments regarding patients while not in a patient's presence, and 38 percent reported hearing the same while in a patient's presence. The task force considered these findings as worrisome and motivating, spurring the group toward efforts to reinforce professionalism throughout the education program at the College of Medicine.

The class of 2001 also completed surveys concerning their previous first-year coursework. Of the second-year students, 97 percent reported a change in attitude for the better toward clinical science faculty and 55 percent better toward colleagues (other students). Fifty-two percent of students reported a change in attitude for the worse toward basic science faculty; 55 percent of this class reported hearing derogatory comments regarding patients while not in a patient's presence with only 3 percent reporting the same while in a patient's presence. Unprofessional conduct of the basic science faculty was observed by 36 percent of students, of the clinical science faculty by 18 percent of students, and of fellow students by 31 percent. These reported changes in attitudes occurring over the span of the previous academic year for both classes of students indicated a pattern of identification of unethical or unprofessional behavior.

Third, using an anonymous responder system during presentations on professionalism to the first-year class, students picked one best answer on a series of questions following four different scenarios. For the entering first-year students, 10–23 percent chose answers deemed inappropriate or characteristic of unprofessional behavior. In one scenario, first-year students watched role playing of a student offering inappropriately obtained answers to another student on a secure exam. Possible choices the students could make on the responder system included not receiving the information, receiving the information and not passing it on, or receiving the information and passing it on. Seventy-seven percent declined the offer, 7 percent would receive the information, and 5 percent would receive and share the information. The remaining 11 percent were unsure of their response.

Entering third-year students were also presented with four scenarios and followup questions. Again using an anonymous responder system, 10–20 percent of students chose inappropriate answers. One role-play example involved an inappropriate dinner invitation from an attending. Here, 75 percent of students refused the offer, 11 percent accepted the offer, and 14 percent were unsure. Student data again identified unprofessional attitudes.

The second source of data for the task force needs assessment came from patients. The Picker Institute, which collects University of Kentucky inpatient satisfaction survey data, found that data collected during August 1996, February 1997, July 1997, and February 1998 revealed that a majority of patients expressed confidence in their doctors, rated the courtesy of their doctors as excellent or very good, rated the availability of their doctors as excellent or very good, and rated their overall care as excellent or very good. There were, however, 11–15 percent of patients who stated the doctors *sometimes* talked in front of them as if they were not there and 2–9 percent who stated the doctors *often* talked in front of them as if they were not there.

The third source of data for the task force needs assessment was faculty and administrators. We surveyed department chairpersons, course directors, and residency directors, asking whether they evaluated and recorded the professional behavior of their faculty and residents. The majority of responders indicated that they did review professional behavior as part of the evaluation process of faculty or residents. They defined "review" as discussing attributes of professional behavior and/or completing evaluation forms on professional behavior. These reviews occurred at regularly scheduled intervals, monthly for residents and yearly for faculty evaluation sessions.

After review of the data from the above sources, the Task Force on Professionalism divided into smaller focus groups to develop suggestions to facilitate the inculcation of professional behavior across the four-year medical school curriculum, as well as to increase awareness and evaluation of professional behavior among resident physicians and faculty. These focus groups included additional medical students, faculty, and administrative staff who had expressed interest in the Professionalism Project after the formation of the original task force. The focus groups submitted the following suggestions to the Task Force on Professionalism:

Medical School Admissions Process. When *recruiting* medical school applicants, the Office of Admissions staff can improve communications regarding professionalism traits when speaking with college advisors; should request letters from community service preceptors to be included in the admissions file; and can conduct pilot studies on peer evaluation of premedical students. As a result of this recommendation, a packet of information is distributed to all premedical advisors emphasizing the importance of professional behavior traits and the relevance of community service. Regarding the *interview* process, suggestions included the use of standardized written cases involving moral reasoning and ethical development, and enhanced training of interviewers on professionalism issues. Finally, in the *acceptance* written materials, the group suggested that a clear statement on professional behavior expectations be included; this statement could be repeated in the student handbook and orientation materials as well as in course syllabi.

Curriculum and Evaluation. The University of Kentucky College of Medicine curriculum is an integrated curriculum in which clinical exposure occurs in basic science courses, and basic science review occurs in clinical clerkships. Across all courses, expectations of professional behavior and a "no tolerance" rule of unprofessional behavior are to be stated more clearly and consistently, both verbally and in written materials. In courses where "paper" patients and "standardized" patients are utilized, learning issues will incorporate professionalism issues and behaviors. Course and clerkship directors should review and update on a recurring basis those cases involving professionalism issues. In the clinical performance examination required at the completion of the third year of medical school, evaluation of professional behavior will be incorporated wherever possible. In addition, the professional code (previously known as the honor code) will be implemented across all medical school years (once university approval is obtained).

In addition, the Testing and Evaluation Office is reviewing data from the professional-behavior section of evaluations and developing summary information to be returned to faculty and students. Institutional Review Board approval has been obtained for a pilot project on a Peer Professional Ratings Program to determine the usefulness of peer evaluations among fourth-year medical students. Finally, positive results will be recognized at all levels of medical school administration: "champions," those displaying the highest professional standards, will be recognized annually at the academic convocation and awards ceremony and their names displayed along with other award winners.

Resident and Faculty Development. This focus group suggested presenting brief, interactive presentations on professionalism issues for resident groups via noon conferences and orientations. Similar presentations will occur for the Council of Chairs group, Community-Based Faculty Continuing Education Meetings, and collegewide faculty meetings. The University of Kentucky Medical Alumni Association will also increase mentoring activities among faculty, alumni, residents, and students. The alumni association is exploring identifying and rewarding "champions" among alumni who demonstrate the highest standards for professional behavior. Finally, the Office of Academic Affairs will identify a group of volunteer ombudspersons who can provide a sounding board for students when ethical questions or professional-behavior dilemmas arise.

These ombudspersons would emphasize the professional behaviors expected of students, residents, and faculty in each situation brought to their attention. Students may have access to this service as a group or on an individual basis. Orientation will occur for those faculty willing to serve.

Extracurricular Activities. The Office of Academic Affairs has developed, organized, or proposed a number of programs to encourage and reward professionalism in medical students. These include a white coat ceremony for entering first-year medical students, an academic convocation and awards ceremony for students and faculty, and class orientations for all students that include presentations on professionalism. A new event planned is "reflections on the white coat ceremony" to occur at the conclusion of third-year clerkships and to honor the professional development of each medical student through an invited speaker, group reflection time, and small-group discussion. Students will receive a pocket-sized notebook from the College of Medicine as a memento and a tool to record future reflections.

———————

The University of Kentucky College of Medicine Professionalism Project has successfully completed a number of recommendations formulated by the focus groups and the task force. Currently, works in progress include a pilot study to develop a bank of moral reasoning cases for use by interviewers in medical school admissions; the fine-tuning of a clinical assessment form to evaluate professional and personal attributes as well as clinical knowledge and skills; selection of the first graduating senior and first faculty member to receive Humanism in Medicine Awards at the 1999 College of Medicine Graduation event; recruiting and orienting of a group of ombudspersons for student questions and concerns regarding professionalism issues; and, finally, execution of the Reflections on the White Coat Ceremony for third-year students completing clinical clerkships. The combination of our history, the working together of our Offices of Academic Affairs and Student Affairs, and small grant monies from the dean's office and the Healthcare Foundation of New Jersey have facilitated this work. Through all these efforts, we believe that medical students progressing through the University of Kentucky College of Medicine will understand the importance of professionalism in all their work.

Sheila Woods, Sue Fosson, and Lois Margaret Nora

JUDITH ANDRE
JAKE FOGLIO
HOWARD BRODY

Moral Growth, Spirituality, and Activism
The Humanities in Medical Education

Thomas Merton points out that being too busy can kill the "root of inner wisdom":

> The rush and pressure of modern life are a form, perhaps the most common form, of its innate violence. . . . The frenzy of the activist neutralizes his work, because it kills the root of inner wisdom which makes work fruitful. (Merton, 1966, p. 86)

Although Merton is referring to political activity, the insight applies even more forcefully to a life in medicine, the demands of which can destroy not only an inner life, but much of an outer one as well; after caring for patients and for one's family, the physician may feel that involvement in the broader community seems impossible. At Michigan State University, the medical school curriculum tries to engage these problems in a variety of ways. While these efforts constitute less than a seamless whole, and we continue to struggle toward something better, some of them are distinctive. We hope the following description of our efforts is of use to others; drawing the strands together has already helped us to articulate more clearly our own basic beliefs.

First, some background: Michigan State University (MSU) has four health care colleges. There are two medical schools — the College of Human Medicine (CHM) and the College of Osteopathic Medicine (COM) — as well as the College of Nursing and the College of Veterinary Medicine. We who teach bioethics and medical humanities work with all four schools, trying different strategies in each; we learn something different in each context. Because the most distinctive part of our curriculum, its "spirituality selective," is offered only in the College of Human Medicine, this article focuses on that college. It is worth noting, however, that the field of osteopathy has a distinctive history. It was founded in 1874 by Andrew Taylor Still, a physician dissatisfied with the prevailing medicine of his day, in particular its reliance on drugs and surgery. In its place, he developed an osteopathic approach to care — one that traced physiological disturbances in the body to abnormalities in the musculoskeletal system. By employing hands-on therapy to correct these structural abnormalities, he believed, physicians could enhance the body's natural tendency toward health and self-healing. (Guglielmo, 1998, p. 201)

For more than a century osteopaths have retained their commitment to primary care, to holistic medicine, and to the importance of the doctor-patient relationship. These are commitments to which allopathic medicine has returned only in the past few decades.

MSU's College of Human Medicine pioneered in that return. Its distinctive history makes it particularly appropriate for the experimental efforts we describe here. Although this essay focuses on CHM, it also draws from our experiences in the College of Osteopathic Medicine and the university's other health care colleges.

––––––––

MSU's College of Human Medicine was founded in 1964, admitted its first students into a two-year curriculum in 1966, and graduated its first M.D.s from a four-year curriculum in 1972. Like many other medical schools founded during that decade, CHM saw itself as marching to a "different drummer," a concept its founding dean Andrew Hunt later used as a conference and book title (Hunt & Weeks, 1979). Many of the new faculty recruited by Hunt were self-described young Turks, who could have advanced by doing scientific or clinical research at prestigious, already established medical schools; instead they were committed to teaching and to finding a better way to train future doctors. MSU itself, a land-grant college which had long defined its mission as service to the people, provided fertile soil for innovation. Work with practical results has always been valued here.

Within its first decade CHM committed itself to the following basic educational values. They are uncontroversial today but seemed radical then:

Fewer lectures, more group discussion
Early exposure to patients
Early training in medical interviewing
Problem-based rather than discipline-based instruction
Inclusion of behavioral and social science material
Training in community hospitals (rather than in a university hospital, which
  we did not and do not have)

Some of the flavor of CHM in its formative days can be heard in a 1997 interview with Peter Ways, one of the first assistant professors hired by the chair of the Department of Medicine, Scott Swisher. Ways helped pioneer two innovations at CHM: first, the "focal problem" curriculum, an early version of what is now called problem-based learning (Ways, Loftus, & Jones, 1973), and second, establishment of a community campus site (in Saginaw) for clinical training. He described this period:

> I'd had a five-year American Heart Association fellowship and an established investigatorship from the Public Health Service, and was known particularly for having made a description of abnormal membrane lipids in red cells . . . so this was big for Swisher, he wanted to bring somebody in who had a strong research program and to build his department in that way. So we packed up these huge gas chromatographs and all kinds of other equipment that I had accumulated over the years and shipped it by van, MSU paid for it. And none of it ever got unpacked by me. I just got too busy doing the educational stuff and setting up the community programs. (Ways, 1997)

Recalling the origin of the focal problem curriculum, he tells how they were

> looking for a way to put the basic sciences into a problem-oriented format so that the students would have an opportunity to . . . ask their own questions, and then answer those questions as part of solving a clinical problem — the clinical problem didn't have to be about an individual, it could be about a community — air pollution or birth control. . . . After my first six months here . . . I had a back operation . . . and suddenly it just sort of bloomed and we went ahead with, I guess then it was our second-year class, they would learn as much or more of their basic science in a focal problem context as in a lecture-oriented context, and that it would also be a format for teaching basic pathophysiology. The most important thing is after the first three — each problem lasted a week, we had the whole class, it was a small class at that time — after the first three or four the students started complaining. We listened to them and they had some ideas about how it might be changed in ways that sounded good. And so the final — I guess it's never been quite final, but — the format that we eventually used for several years had a very significant student input. (Ways, 1997)

This story highlights some basic features of CHM in those years. At the time a very junior faculty member, Ways had the authority to redesign a major portion of the medicine curriculum. He imagined the new curricular design while in bed recovering from surgery, and within a few weeks his ideas were being tried out — amazing speed from today's perspective where (in CHM as elsewhere) a great new idea might be proposed and, with luck, be approved by all the relevant committees and gingerly pilot-tested after a mere two or three years' consideration. Finally, the faculty of that day saw themselves fundamentally as allies and partners of the medical students; they prized an egalitarian environment in which students as well as the faculty could influence the college.

CHM came into being, of course, at a time when the country was filled with energy and unrest: the civil rights, antiwar, environmental, and women's movements filled newspapers, living rooms, and sometimes the streets, and much of it was shaped by student activism. CHM retains an enduring and pervasive sense that it exists, in part, to train physicians who will be leaders in their communities, who take seriously the college motto, "Serving the People." Several aspects of CHM in the 1970s suggest the nature and origins of that commitment. Many early faculty members saw themselves as visionaries battling with the forces of reaction — with established medical schools and, most particularly, with the Liaison Committee on Medical Education (LCME), which had the power to bestow or refuse accreditation. The LCME would have preferred that CHM adopt a low profile appropriate to its neophyte status: that is, require its students to take standardized tests; establish a conventional curriculum; and then, slowly and cautiously, begin experimenting with the curriculum. CHM rather openly showed its contempt for the standardized measures of educational merit, and in some instances almost dared the LCME to take away its accreditation. The most notable case was the Upper Peninsula project, in which CHM proposed to train a small group of students for their entire four years at a family health center in Escanaba, hundreds of miles north of the main campus. After several years of pitched battle with the LCME under Hunt and his successor, Donald Weston, CHM was finally forced to close down the preclinical aspect of the project and to require all students to pass the standard board exams (Heagerty, n.d.).

Medical ethics and medical humanities were not initially part of CHM's mission. (Its name, College of Human Medicine, was chosen to distinguish the school from the College of Veterinary Medicine, not from any explicit commitment to humanities or humanism.) When, however, a national movement toward including ethics and humanities gathered steam in the early 1970s, CHM faculty responded with enthusiasm. They had built a school open to such innovations: its treatment of the physician-patient relationship as a human interaction and its preference for seminars over lectures provided a

Judith Andre, Jake Foglio, and Howard Brody

natural welcome for ethics discussion; the faculty's inclusion of social and behavioral scientists created a tradition of interdisciplinary collaboration. When Hunt left the deanship in 1977, he became the founding director of the Medical Humanities Program, later the Center for Ethics and Humanities in the Life Sciences (Hunt & Brody, 1983). By 1981 an ethics course was a required part of the second-year curriculum, and in 1992 a short required course in humanities was added.

By the early 1990s, however, the world and CHM had changed. Until then the faculty had not seen cheating as a problem: our pass-fail grading system and small-group instructional format encouraged cooperative learning rather than competition; perhaps faculty also thought their admissions interviews excluded "that sort" of student in the first place. Like other medical schools at the time (Anderson & Obenshian, 1994), CHM awakened to the knowledge that cheating was an important problem requiring explicit solutions.

––––––––

In 1994, Ruth Hoppe, associate dean for academic programs, created the Task Force on Professional Behavior to address the issue. To its credit, the task force defined its mission broadly. It sought not just to reduce cheating on exams, but also to incorporate the effective teaching of professional behavior throughout the curriculum. The task force believed it should scrutinize faculty and staff as well as students, since professional values ought to be evident in the way courses are taught and the school is organized. For example, if students are expected to "turn in" someone who cheats on an exam, perhaps they should also be expected to turn in faculty who are poor role models in the classroom or clinic. And the school should provide a safe environment for students who accept this responsibility.

When the task force looked through the curriculum for resources that would help with their task, it did not find the ethics course particularly useful, but it found another humanities component quite promising. Toward the end of their second year, all students spend eight classroom hours studying one of three humanities modules — Spirituality and Medicine, History and Medicine, or Literature and Medicine. The spirituality selective caught the task force's attention.

We want to explain and affirm their sense that spirituality, more than conventional ethics teaching, grounds the deepest thinking about the person — the physician — that one wants to become. But we will also argue that ethics courses are not irrelevant to this project, even in their most conventional form, and that interesting things can be done to make ethics courses more relevant to personal and professional development.

First, some theoretical considerations. We think of "professional development" as including moral development — or, in the terms we prefer, moral growth. Each of these phrases is a technical term, clear to those immersed in its literature, more opaque to those who are not. "Moral development" has particular difficulties: first, developmental theories tend to assume universal and invariant stages of development. No stage can be skipped; everyone everywhere goes from the first to the second, only then to the third, and so on. This means that developmental models carry heavy and contestable theoretical baggage. Secondly, the pioneering work in moral development was done by Lawrence Kohlberg (1984), who equated it with progress in moral judgment.

We prefer the term *moral growth* to moral development because the former is less technical and more open. It allows for many different dimensions and patterns of growth. For one thing, as James Rest (1982) points out, people vary greatly in their ability to recognize the needs of others: the most sophisticated reasoning will not help someone who has no questions. Human beings grow not only in reasoning but also in moral perception, and in what Rest calls "ego strength" — the ability actually to do what one has decided is right. Furthermore these three — perception, judgment, and strength of character — do not exhaust the dimensions in which one can grow morally. Relationships, for instance, may be more or less moral; virtues, with their constellation of understanding, feeling, and habitual action, are gained and lost through time. Even "reasoning" should be understood more broadly than Kohlberg did: it is not just a matter of making difficult decisions, but also of something less schematic. Moral reflection, progress in moral understanding, takes many different forms.

————

Following earlier work by one of us (Andre, 1991), we find it useful to think of moral growth as concerned with at least three objects: oneself, others (as individuals), and social systems. Growth is a matter of deepening one's understanding of what is of value (human beings deserve respect that tissue does not), and of learning to respond appropriately to what one understands. Appropriate responses demand more than reasoning: they require supportive habits and a variety of skills; often they require courage, usually wisdom as well — and more. We will be speaking of moral growth, then, as a matter of becoming more able to see and to respond appropriately to what is of value, in individuals (including oneself) and in human systems. We offer this account not as an exhaustive description of what is involved in moral growth, but as a broad and practical approach to the question.

Against that background, where does formal ethics teaching fit? The course we teach in CHM has been a rigorous, case-centered (and usually dilemma-centered) coverage of central issues in academic medical ethics. In one sense it focuses on Kohlbergian "moral judgment," and encourages students to reach more reasoned stands on hard cases (refusal of life-saving treatment, for instance, or physician-assisted suicide). These tend to be dramatic, end-of-life issues. Other aspects of the course, however, contribute to moral growth in the wider sense that we propose here. The texts, for one thing, are not all "straight bioethics." We include literature and social science, both of which help students think in broader ways about patients, themselves, and the world. Furthermore, as we all know, the medium is (part of) the message, and the fact that the course is conducted entirely in small groups (eight to ten students) is significant. Students are graded (pass-fail) on their participation in the small groups, and gain important practice in respectful conversation about ethical matters. Each of us has seen, for instance, students whose views are unusual (religious fundamentalists, or political extremists) welcomed and respected within a discussion. This is no accident: the culture of CHM small groups encourages it, as does the deliberately diverse admissions policy, and the carefully worked out statement in our syllabus addressing the role of religion within a pluralist discussion.

Context is also part of instruction, and here the contrast between the two medical schools on the one hand and the College of Veterinary Medicine on the other is striking. All these schools have conscientious faculty, good clinicians in every sense. But *medical* ethics has been part of the public culture for decades now, as veterinary ethics has not, and the results are significant. Medical students tend to realize that there is some point to ethical reading and conversation. They are far less likely than veterinary students to be stuck in "naive relativism" — the a priori rejection of moral reasoning as pointless ("But that's a value judgment!" or, "Who's to say what's right and wrong?"). The American context encourages serious reflection about medical ethics, as does the culture of CHM.

For all these reasons we hope that our ethics course in CHM, through its content, context, and structure, contributes to moral growth widely construed. We realize, however, that a formal ethics course could deal with moral growth more widely than ours does now. In fact our most innovative activity takes place in the other college, the osteopathic school, in a course designed by our colleague Tom Tomlinson. Its final unit concerns "bad outcomes" and integrates a broad range of materials on doctors' mistakes. The readings include Lucien L. Leape (1994) on systems analysis, David Hilfiker's personal essay on mistakes (1987), and material about malpractice (meant to relieve some of the exaggerated fears that are prevalent and to commend doctors who put patients' interests ahead of legal worries).

———

These readings and lectures set the stage for a radical final session: a panel in which three or four physicians discuss their own mistakes — serious ones. The session fosters something that, as Leape and Hilfiker so powerfully point out, is missing in medical culture: a space for admitting one's mistakes, putting them in perspective, dealing with them. Fostering such a space, we hope, contributes to moral growth in its broadest sense. The panel helps students develop a more realistic sense of themselves and their colleagues and demonstrates healthier ways of dealing with fallibility. When error is suppressed — and this seems to be the medical norm — underlying causes cannot be dealt with, and the individual doctor is likely to suffer greatly. That suffering will never be eliminated, nor should it be. But in the wrong form it is more likely to cripple than to transform.

Our thoughts about what a formal ethics course can accomplish are also shaped somewhat by our contacts with msu's College of Nursing. Nurses face the same kind of dilemmas doctors do, but they face them from quite a different stance. The difference most relevant to this paper is one of power. Because they have so much less authority, nurses often suffer from what Jameton and Wilkinson (1993) call "moral distress." This is a problem different from the dilemmas with which bioethics more often deals: "moral distress" occurs when one knows what should be done but is powerless to bring it about; ordinarily one feels in some way complicit, as part of the system (or "team") that one believes is mistreating a patient. Although this experience was first identified (as far as we know) in the nursing literature, it is common elsewhere. Medical students and residents are also relatively powerless. And the current corporatizing of medicine makes many senior physicians feel the same way. One of the lessons to be learned from nursing's longstanding discussion of the issue is that moral action demands more than good reasoning: it requires courage, discretion, and skill in speaking out. Furthermore it demands collective action.

We incorporate at least one of these lessons in our third-year chm ethics sessions, whose only required readings concern the challenges of the medical student role: "Primum non tacere" — above all, do not keep silent (Dwyer, 1994). This is easy to say, of course, but hard to live by. So we end our third-year sessions by having students present cases to the hospital ethics committee, hoping that the exercise prepares them to make use of ethics committees throughout their careers. We may also try to acquaint them with other hospital resources, from quality control through risk management and patient support. The point,

Judith Andre, Jake Foglio, and Howard Brody

again, is that ethical action requires more than figuring out what should be done, hard and important as that is; it also requires knowing how to get it done.

At times this demands working together, not just as a "health care team," but also as groups with political agendas. We are social animals: by nature we live together in orderly ways. Societies are sets of systems, formal and informal. Bioethics scholarship has begun to deal with systems issues, looking at the once neglected problems that lie between individual choices and societal decisions. One of us has written on the ways in which managed care plans can be good or bad (Clancy & Brody, 1995). Haavi Morreim, a recent invited speaker, led us through an exercise about a death that resulted from the fantastic complexity of structures within health care today: HMO regulations, practice agreements, incentive structures, state law, and so on and so on (see Crigger, 1998). The point which social scientists made in vain for many years is finally clear throughout bioethics: systems are important. We are beginning to try to draw the moral corollary: an ethical life must be at times a political one.

––––––––

An ethical life, then, demands the full use of human capacities. Gradually we are shaping our various ethics courses so that they contribute more fully to this kind of development. Reasoning, of course, remains central. But we understand reason, too, in a somewhat broader way than do many; we do not see it as simply a matter of calculation. Cognitive science now distinguishes many different ways in which the mind interacts with and makes sense of the world. For our part we would like to flag what we call reflection. The spirituality selective offers to second-year students our best means of encouraging that.

Teaching Spirituality: Reflection and Praxis

The Task Force on Professional Behavior at CHM saw the relatively new spirituality selective as one of the school's most promising resources. In large part this was because it is one of the few formal opportunities within the college encouraging sustained self-reflection. Because the course is unusual, perhaps even unique, we will describe it in some detail.

Developing the course required moving beyond the vagueness often associated with spirituality. As we use it, spirituality refers to one's orientation toward such supreme values as love, meaning, beauty, hope, and truth. One's values and purposes; one's conception of peace, compassion, and personhood; one's understanding of death and grieving; simple self-reflection — all these are also expressions of spirituality.

This conception of spirituality makes it a universal feature of being human, and not the same thing as being religious. Secular, religious, atheist, and agnostic spiritualities are all possible and worthy of respect. James Bacik (1996) describes spirituality as "a search for meaning in the midst of absurdity, for integration that overcomes fragmentation, for depth in a culture which fosters superficiality, for purpose in an often directionless world," and notes that many participate in this spiritual search without any direct relationship to religion (p. 6). Whatever the form of their spirituality, medical students need support and guidance in the task of becoming the physicians they hope to become.

Briefly put, spirituality is the search for what ultimately gives meaning to life. This search is of special importance within medicine, because much of the suffering that accompanies serious disease is produced by, and can only be alleviated through, the personal meaning one attaches to the experience (Cassell, 1991). Reflecting upon existence in the Auschwitz concentration camp, Victor Frankl (1959) claimed that often the difference between those who survived and those who died was that the former found a way to construct meaning for their lives, even under those terrible circumstances. Giving meaning to one's experiences — understanding them in the light of one's deepest values — appears to be vital to human well-being. Helping students discern these fundamental values as they shape meaningful professional and personal lives is what the spirituality curriculum is all about.

Many thinkers have tried to relate spirituality to the biopsychosocial model, which has become a popular heuristic for the "modern" medical curriculum. We prefer the view of Hiatt (1986) and Carr (1994), who point out that for all its strengths the biopsychosocial model lacks an overall integrating framework. The spiritual dimension ought to be identified with that integrating framework and not with any specific "level" of systems functioning within the model itself. Thus, our proposal is not for a "bio-psycho-social-spiritual" model to replace the original formulation. Rather, the biological, psychological, and social dimensions of one's life are all aspects of spirituality.

———

As Buxbaum (1997) points out, too often people define spirituality as a pious withdrawal from life; instead it should be seen as the courage to find meaning in full engagement with life. The resemblance between this concept of spirituality and what we referred to earlier as moral growth is striking. The difference, perhaps, is one of emphasis: spiritual growth more clearly demands a habit of reflection. In other words, our understanding of moral development is richer than

Judith Andre, Jake Foglio, and Howard Brody

the one found in the psychological literature, and our understanding of spirituality fuller than that in popular culture. Each involves more aspects of a human being than has been customary. It is not surprising that the two conceptions overlap.

Nevertheless the two courses — ethics and spirituality — are quite distinct. The ethics course concentrates on fairly explicit reasoning, especially public reasoning; the spirituality module offers tools for a different and more personal kind of work. Virtue involves not only habitual action but also the habit of reflection: a regular consideration of personal values and meanings, and of the fit between one's life and those underlying values. Spiritual reflection is something like physical exercise — just as everyone (including physicians) needs bodily exercise for optimal health, regular time and energy devoted to reflection are essential for spiritual well-being. Finding the time and energy for both sorts of exercise often means getting beyond the "busyness" of daily life — which, as Stephen R. Covey (1989) has pointed out, can keep us from distinguishing between the urgent and the important. Much of what seems urgent has little ultimate significance.

Thomas Merton, with whose words we began this essay, understood the problem. Here is the full quotation:

> There is a pervasive form of contemporary violence to which the idealist, fighting for peace by nonviolent methods, most easily succumbs: activism and overwork. The rush and pressure of modern life are a form, perhaps the most common form, of its innate violence. To allow oneself to be carried away by a multitude of conflicting concerns, to surrender to too many demands. To commit oneself to too many projects, to want to help everyone in everything is to succumb to violence. The frenzy of the activist neutralizes his work, because it kills the root of inner wisdom which makes work fruitful. (1986, p. 86)

Merton was himself what most would describe as an activist in the antiwar movement of the 1960s. Yet in this passage he identifies both the daily lives of many activists, and the personal habits of almost all modern physicians, as a way of participating in violence against human values, rather than ways of promoting peace and health.

The spirituality course not only makes this point, but offers a set of concepts and practices to help students gain balance in their own lives. For many students the most important distinction offered is that between chronological or "clock" time, on the one hand, and contemplative time on the other. Relying solely on the first and devaluing the second pushes otherwise laudable impulses — for example, to serve others — into the realm of violence. The reading which seems to make the most lasting impression describes the difference between the two Greek words for time. While *chronos* refers to what can be measured by the clock or calendar, *kairos* refers instead to time that cannot be measured, time that is separated instead into periods of meaning. In reflection one temporarily steps outside of chronological time to see things from a different level and with a more broadly purposeful perspective (Bloomquist, 1997). In many ways the distinction between *chronos* and *kairos* parallels Covey's distinction between the urgent and the important. Helping students learn to value *kairos* in their lives, and to resist being swallowed by *chronos*, is a critical goal of spirituality teaching.

We describe a variety of exercises as aids in regular reflection. These include transcendental and other forms of meditation, yoga, relaxation response, contemplation, and journaling. Each is a means toward an inward focus, a way to find space within oneself despite a culture so much at odds with it. The intensity and sensory overstimulation of contemporary life almost deny the reality of anything quieter. Again, however, the course does not encourage spirituality as an escape from the world. On the contrary: an inner life is part of, and nourishes, a full and balanced life.

Some of the course uses concepts from academic ethics, but it chooses those that deal with personal qualities rather than with the rightness of one's choices. We talk about character, integrity, and conscience, for instance, and about learning how to love. Integrity, with its implication of wholeness, is especially appropriate here, since we conceive of spirituality as an integrating framework (Benjamin, 1990). Integrity by itself does not assure that the values chosen to shape one's attitudes and behavior will be good ones; one must appeal to some system of ethics to establish the moral correctness of those values — hence, again, the interdependence of ethics and spirituality. And again it is important to do, not just think; only practice can make behavior in accord with one's core values habitual, while at the same time challenging and refining one's understanding of those values. Here the course cites MacIntyre (1981): acting virtuously means striving for a kind of excellence in one's actions and behavior; like other excellences in difficult, complex activities, moral virtue demands continuous practice.

The course also takes up questions of special importance in medicine: the possible meanings of suffering, the role a patient's spirituality plays in his or her experience of illness, and some ways a physician may appropriately work with that orientation. The medical curriculum emphasizes scientific and technical skills, and stresses that, without continuing education, physicians become unable to care for their patients. Practice is needed for technical skills — even the best physicians soon become rusty if they do not do a procedure for a while. The humane skills that constitute virtuous behavior — such things as imparting hope, and showing compassion through intensive listening — likewise require practice. The physician's ability to promote healing depends on both sets of skills. Covey (1989) has shrewdly observed that ability and character tend to go together; allowing one's abilities to atrophy through inadequate practice commonly reflects a character flaw. And, as Richard Gula notes, "We must practice virtuous activity so that the virtues become habits, or second nature to us. We become trustworthy by doing acts of trustworthiness; we become altruistic by doing acts of altruism" (1996, p. 20).

Medical ethics as routinely taught in U.S. medical schools can help students discern what counts as a good decision in a particular case, and which general principles might lead to better decisions being made. But ethics teaching often does not address the process of becoming a professional while remaining a whole person — one whose personal values blend with the ideals of excellent professional practice, and whose professional practice embodies and demonstrates one's fully developed human excellences. A spirituality course can supplement an ethics course in important ways toward this goal, but no single, limited course is sufficient. Ideally the entire four-year curriculum, as well as the faculty who serve as role models, will demonstrate the amalgam of analytic thought, sustained reflection, and daily praxis that supports the development of professional virtue. Rob Lehman (president of the Fetzer Institute, which has supported a number of spirituality initiatives in medicine) summarized the principal reason for teaching in this way: "We come with the belief that, when we see clearly, we will discover what the great spiritual traditions have taught, and that is, simply, as we enhance our inner capacity for wholeness and freedom, we strengthen our capacity to love and serve" (1998, p. 1).

While CHM has throughout its brief history prided itself on trying to be a different sort of place, humility and realism require us to be skeptical about the degree of difference that actually exists, especially between CHM and other medical schools that train students in community hospitals. Unfortunately, what our graduates learn in residency probably influences them more strongly than most of what transpires in their undergraduate medical years. Still, two studies have shown significant differences between CHM students and those in the other Michigan allopathic schools — that CHM students value ethics and humanism considerably more highly (Maheux & Beland, 1986; Herzberg, 1998) — and we also hear informally that our graduates are superior in this regard. Nevertheless, we know of no real data showing that the attitudinal differences persist over the years.

It does seem reasonable to propose, however, that CHM's foundational aspirations to train activist physicians had an important if subtle influence on the academic environment, which welcomed the courses in ethics and spirituality and shaped the way in which they are taught. In addition, while some might view a curriculum which tries to stress moral reflection as passive (and therefore as contrary to the goal of activism), we have tried to show, through an account of moral growth, that the two are integrally connected and mutually supportive.

Judith Andre, Jake Foglio, and Howard Brody

MARY ANNE C. JOHNSTON

Reflections on Experiences with Socially Active Students

As faculty in medical schools debate the best ways to teach professional and ethical behaviors to students, medical students have acted to develop their own professional skills. As an educator in three medical schools for the past twelve years, I have had an opportunity to work with students and faculty as they create formal curricula and educational programs that address the needs for professional development of both groups. This chapter will describe some personal experiences with students who have taken responsibility for their own professional development. I will narrate the stories of students who have exhibited active leadership in promoting their own and other students' professional development.

Physicians have always prided themselves on a sense of professionalism that is fundamental to the practice of medicine. Many physician groups and medical organizations are now interested in delineating the characteristics of the professional in the practice of medicine. The American Board of Internal Medicine recently published the document *Project Professionalism* to address the importance of professionalism in medicine (ABIM, 1995). It states that "professionalism in medicine requires the physician to serve the interest of the patient above his or her self-interest. Professionalism *aspires* to altruism, accountability, excellence, duty, service, honor, integrity and respect for others" (p. 5). Moreover, the elements of professionalism for their board candidates include "a commitment to the highest standards of excellence in the practice of medicine and in the generation and dissemination of knowledge, a commitment to sustain the interests and welfare of patients, and a commitment to be responsive to the health needs of society" (p. 5). In addition, the ABIM (1992) also created a guide with detailed definitions and case studies to assist faculty in promoting the development of humanistic behaviors, an important component of professionalism, in residents and subspecialty fellows.

In the Medical Schools Objectives Project, the Association of American Medical Colleges (1998) recently developed a proposal for medical educators that defines the goals and objectives of medical education. The goals are described as a series of professional attributes (altruistic, knowledgeable, skillful, dutiful) that medical students should possess in order "to meet their individual and collective responsibilities to society" (p. 6). This proposal lists broad learning objectives under each professional attribute. Medical schools are encouraged to use these objectives to guide them in creating learning objectives for their own medical students.

Finally, a group of highly respected physician-educators issued a "patient-physician covenant" (Crawshaw et al., 1995) to reiterate their definition of professionalism during the rapid changes in health care during the past decade. They wrote,

> Medicine is, at its center, a moral enterprise grounded in a covenant of trust. This covenant obliges physicians to be competent and to use their competence in the patient's best interests. Physicians, therefore, are both intellectually and morally obliged to act as advocates for the sick wherever their welfare is threatened and for their health at all times. . . . Only by caring and advocating for the patient can the integrity of our profession be affirmed. Thus we honor our covenant of trust with patients. (p. 1553)

Students themselves are grappling with the definitions of professionalism in an age when static conceptions of "core values" may not lead to the development of such values or attributes in medical students. Feudtner and Christakis (1994) contend that "medical ethics education must consider the meandering and arduous journey that students make on their way to becoming ethical physicians — that the nature of this odyssey will shape the kind of doctors they will become" (p. 11).

The public has also become interested in what it means to be a professional in medicine today. In the new world of managed care, there is sometimes uncertainty about the role and responsibility of physicians. The AAMC (Cohen, 1999a) recently questioned eight hundred Americans to identify traits they would seek in the selection of a doctor: "Eighty-five percent wanted their doctor to communicate and to have a caring attitude; 76% wanted their doctor to take the time to listen to them; 77% wanted their doctor to explain things in a way they could understand" (p. 109).

Although there will be continued debate on exactly what professionalism means to various constituents of our society, medical schools will need to address the task of preparing their students to be professionals in medicine. As medical schools strive to identify the values, attributes, and behaviors that reflect the "good physician," it is likely to be even more difficult to determine how to promote their development in students. In the following pages, I propose that medical students themselves are keenly invested in professionalism and, in an environment that fosters student intiative, can become vital sources for their own professional growth.

———

A small group of first- and second-year students initiated a major change in the required curriculum at Yale in the spring of 1994. These students asked to speak to the Educational Policy and Curriculum Committee (EPCC) to present their concerns about the lack of sensitivity among their peers and faculty to diverse populations, especially on issues related to ethnicity and sexual orientation. Some students were concerned about insensitive classes, instructors, and visual aids. In addition, the medical students discussed their frustrations regarding the lack of content on health data related to different cultural groups in the medical school curriculum at Yale.

In response to these concerns, the EPCC formed the Committee on Multicultural Education to investigate ways to incorporate multicultural and diversity issues into the medical school curriculum. In addition to assessing the degree to which these issues were presently being addressed in the curriculum, the committee was asked to recommend strategies to increase students' understanding of the health concerns and behaviors of culturally diverse populations. Members of this committee included six self-selected students, three faculty members, the associate dean of curriculum, and the director of the Office of Education. The committee met every other week throughout the fall of 1994. The committee initially examined the content of several major courses to determine the adequacy of information on diverse populations. After several weeks of review, members of the committee decided to construct a course that would increase students' understanding in this area.

A five-week pilot module was created to promote the development of knowledge, skills, and attitudes that would heighten the students' ability to care for any person, regardless of differences in age, culture, ethnicity, gender, physical characteristics, race, religion, sexual orientation, or socioeconomic status. The goals of the multicultural course are to recognize the cultural differences that may affect the health concerns of patients and to identify communications skills that promote understanding and respect for differences. Following an introductory lecture, students participate in four one-and-one-half-hour small-group sessions with selected faculty as facilitators. The students present clinical case studies to facilitate discussion of the physician's role and responsibility in providing health care for individuals from different population groups. The clinical case studies also touch on the issues of religion, complementary medicine, linguistic barriers/interpretation, and reproductive choices. Students often choose role playing and other exercises to promote interaction among themselves.

This new curricular program would not have been designed without the assertiveness and persistence of a small group of students. As much as the faculty wanted to create more opportunities for students to work with diverse populations of patients, it took student commitment to begin the arduous task of constructing an effective program to heighten professional understanding and skills. One student was so enthusiastic about this program that she initiated the writing of a descriptive piece for publication (Gupta, Duffy, & Johnston, 1997).

———

At the University of Pennsylvania, I worked with many students who stepped forward with concerns about professionalism, or the lack of professionalism, as experienced at the medical school. Two fourth-year students volunteered to present the ethics course for third-year students in the required medicine clerkship. They became concerned that the topics in the course dealt with major biomedical issues (transplantation, physician-assisted suicide), whereas the students were struggling with personal ethical dilemmas in their daily interactions with patients and their clinician colleagues. They approached the course director with a request to include a series of ethical seminars called "ward ethics" to address these challenges. Students were encouraged to bring cases that they had personally encountered during their clerkship. The cases were used to promote reflection upon their thoughts and feelings about these experiences. As a final task, students were asked to write a two-page case report on an ethical problem with which they had struggled.

The two fourth-year students shared with me and others at the school a paper in which they described the ethical dilemmas that students faced in their clerkships and the curriculum they developed to address these. This paper (Christakis & Feudtner, 1993) developed into a publication that has influenced other faculty and students who are interested in the ethical development of students and residents.

They also designed studies to investigate the extent of ethical dilemmas faced by students during their clerkship experiences. They were interested not only in the types of dilemmas that medical students believed they encountered, but their feelings about these experiences and whether these dilemmas had influenced their ethical development. The report on their studies (Feudtner, Christakis, &

Mary Anne C. Johnston

Christakis, 1994) has been presented at conferences and published. Since graduation, these physicians have continued to speak out on the significance of providing opportunities for students and residents to deal with their own personal ethical dilemmas. One of their recommendations is especially helpful in creating educational programs in professional development today:

> By attending to the experiences, high and low, that make up the daily rounds of clinical clerks, and by caring as much about their ethical as their intellectual development, perhaps medical education could help students to complete the journey with their humanity and compassion intact. (Feudtner & Christakis, 1994, p. 11)

————

"Day 4: YMS 2000 Warmup" was the title of the four-hour experience that second-year medical students created for incoming students during orientation week at Yale in 1996. During the previous five months, one second-year student coordinated the efforts of over one-third of the second-year students to design a program that would help new students become comfortable with one another in a medical school environment. The general purposes were stated as follows: "[to offer] a formal welcome from the second-year class to the first-year class; an opportunity for team building and trust building; a chance for the first- and second-year classes to meet and 'bond'; and a structured way for members of the first-year class to meet each another." Interactive exercises were created to promote collegiality and respect among students. The small-group interviews, a visualization activity, and a cultural game called BaFa BaFa were the most effective exercises, as judged by the first-year students. In the visualization exercise, students are guided to imagine the experience of meeting their first patients. During the BaFa BaFa game, students are divided into two groups with different norms and behaviors and then asked to interact with one another. What may have been most remarkable about this process was the excitement generated by the upper-class students in welcoming new students into their community.

This orientation experience has evolved over the six years since a second-year student expressed concern that the diversity training that had been offered during orientation at Yale in 1992 failed to deal with issues related to all ethnic and cultural differences. The major focus had been on discrimination among racial groups in the United States. She wanted to broaden the discussion to differences in religion, ethnicity, and sexual orientation. The students who have planned this orientation activity every year since 1993 have expended amazing energy and enthusiasm on a topic that is often given short shrift. Faculty and staff have given educational support and advice only when requested.

Students may best convey the message that respect for diversity is an important concern at the medical center. Even with the best intentions, presentations by faculty and staff can be perceived as preachy and patronizing. A moralizing tone can create even more resistance to thinking constructively about these issues. If the goal during orientation is to increase first-year students' comfort in thinking and talking about diversity, it is probably more helpful to have upper-class students facilitate this process.

This program has also been beneficial to upper-class students. Students who take responsibility for creating and implementing an educational program for their colleagues are likely to become empowered to speak out on ethical and professional issues that will confront them throughout their medical careers. As each of us (faculty and students) learns to communicate our beliefs, thoughts, and feelings, we increase our understanding of commonalities as well as differences. As we begin to understand one another, we are more likely to create a collegial environment that promotes mutual trust and respect.

I experienced another situation in which a group of students became concerned over perceived unprofessional behaviors by faculty toward women and minority students within the classroom setting. After their first year at the University of Pennsylvania School of Medicine in 1989, a self-selected group of students, diverse as to gender, age, ethnicity, and sexual orientation, were alarmed not only by faculty behavior but also by negative interactions between the students themselves, reflecting thoughtlessness and disdain toward differences. After discussions with school administrators, the students were encouraged to share their concerns with their classmates. During a special class meeting for second-year students, the students presented a moving report on the issues as they viewed them, and they reenacted examples of unprofessional behavior. The program resulted in a great deal of thoughtful discussion of the severity of the problem and strategies to handle insensitive behaviors.

In order to respond further to the concerns of the students, the Office of Educational Development decided to provide similar programs for the faculty. We believed that the faculty would benefit from educational experiences that would heighten their own sensitivity to diversity. To stimulate their interest, we created a highly interactive, experiential seminar. In a two-hour workshop format, we used video, role playing, discussion, and small-group activities to maximize the involvement and interaction among the participants.

We decided that a video that gave specific examples of insensitive behavior would present the concerns of medical students most vividly. The students were responsible for making the video, illustrating their own experiences with insensitive or inappropriate behaviors. Some examples follow:

Three African American students are beginning a new clinical clerkship. The attending physician sees her students for the first time at the orientation session. Her initial response is, "Well, if it isn't Gladys Knight and the Pips."

One of the male anatomy professors who has been extremely helpful to an anatomy group of four women students excitedly mentions that he wants to show them the appendix. When the professor shows them the inchworm-sized organ, one woman exclaims, "That's it? That's all there is? But it is so small." The professor smiles, steps back, and calls over several other students to the group. He then asks her to repeat what she has said, which she dutifully does. After her comment, he says, "Boy, you're going to be one tough cookie to please. I would hate to be your husband come honeymoon night. That's it; that's all there is!"

In the operating room, a resident mentions that he thinks a medical student is gay. The faculty surgeon responds, "Just don't let that fag in my OR. It takes long enough to teach a normal student how to catheterize a patient."

The video took almost a year to make. The Office of Educational Development provided guidance and the modest financial support needed. A total of eighteen students were involved in developing, editing, rehearsing, and filming the vignettes. The students said that creating this video was a powerful learning experience for them. Not only did they construct an impressive piece of work that addresses critical issues in the professional development of physicians, they also expanded their understanding of the different values, beliefs, and behaviors among their colleagues. This workshop on increasing skills in working with diverse populations has been provided to faculty members, residents, and students. The voices of the students in the role-playing vignettes are a provocative stimulus for reflecting upon the values and behaviors of a medical professional (Johnston, 1992).

———

Another socially active student took responsibility for changing the learning environment for himself and others by taking another path. His story begins during his first year at Yale School of Medicine in 1992. He became increasingly aware of homophobic behavior on the part of his own classmates, including a comment written at the bottom of an AIDS-awareness poster, placed in the elevator of the medical school dormitory, with an illustration of two men. The handwritten comment placed on the poster said:

Law of Darwinism / Survival of Fittest:
If you can't / won't pass on your genes
then nature will kill you off.

The student brought several such incidents to the attention of the associate dean for student affairs and education. Knowing my interest in increasing sensitivity to diversity, the dean shared several of the student's letters with me, without identifying the student.

However, in the beginning of the student's second year, I presented a workshop on how to handle inappropriate behaviors or comments regarding homosexuality at a meeting of the Lambda Health Alliance (a gay, lesbian, and bisexual group of students and faculty). In this workshop, I used the above incident as one of the cases for discussion and role playing. At that time, a student disclosed that he had been the one to report this behavior.

In January of his second year, during a human sexuality colloquium, the student spoke with his classmates of his personal experiences as a gay man. His reflections on this event demonstrate the value of communicating one's thoughts and feelings to others:

> Over three semesters, I had come out to several classmates, the dean, and our chaplain, like a cautious swimmer who sticks his toes in the river to feel the temperature and the strength of the undertow. As I contemplated jumping in with both feet, I considered the impact I could have on my colleagues, the freedom I would gain to express myself openly and honestly, and the foundation I would establish upon which to continue promoting tolerance and understanding. My only anxiety was, would I appear confident in my presentation? . . . As I reflect on the feeling of leaving the stage to thunderous applause and a swell of emotional and supportive classmates around me, I realize the magnitude of what I have done for them and for myself. By taking this confident step toward becoming an openly gay physician, the "leader by example" that I want so very much to be, I have earned the respect of my peers, who admire my courage, ask questions to increase their understanding, and thank me for making sensitivity to sexual orientation have personal meaning in their lives. (Personal communication, 1993)

Several months later, this student decided that the Yale physician's oath, adapted from the Hippocratic oath, needed to be changed. He wanted to include "sexual orientation" as well as "gender" in the nondiscrimination statement. He discussed this with several administrators and in 1994, for the first time, graduating seniors at Yale read this statement as a part of their oath: "I will not permit considerations of *gender*, race, religion, *sexual orientation*, nationality, or social standing to influence my duty to care for those in need of my service" (emphasis added). Again reaching out to his colleague-students, he along with all of the class officers wrote an open letter to all medical students to communicate the rationale for this change. The letter read in part:

> No matter what specialty we choose, we will be responsible for the health of gay, lesbian, and bisexual people; pediatricians will treat the children of gay patients, obstetricians will deliver babies of lesbian couples, psychiatrists will help teenagers who are struggling with issues of sexual orientation, internists will care for those afflicted with HIV infection, etc. In addition, all of us will care for gay, lesbian, and bisexual patients for whom sexual orientation is irrelevant to their health problems but is vital to their social identity and sense of well-being. (Yale oath, 1994, p. 43)

This student has had tremendous influence on the changes that are occurring at Yale. It has been highly satisfying to work with someone who communicates so honestly and compassionately. As an educator, I am convinced that nothing is more critical to the change process than the ability to communicate.

My experiences with activist students remind me of the quote attributed to Margaret Mead: "Never doubt that a small group of thoughtful, committed citizens can change the world; indeed, it is the only thing that ever has." As I reflect upon my years working with medical students, I would go further and suggest that every person has the opportunity to change her or his own world, no matter how narrow or wide that world might appear to be. We each have the power to create an environment that enhances our personal and professional development, and this, in turn, may enhance the personal and professional development of others.

What I Have Learned

Students who are activists in their own professional development can be exceptional role models for other students, as well as faculty. One student or a small group of students can be especially effective in constructing meaningful educational programs for themselves and their colleagues, as well as faculty. We should support these students as they seek to participate in or create educational programs that enhance professionalism.

Current understanding of how adults learn dictates that in developing curriculum for professionalism, faculty need to involve students actively in experiences that call for engagement and reflection. Faculty are more effective when they listen and respond to students' expressed needs. Students often know what they need in order to develop professional values, traits, and skills.

Communication is an essential skill in the practice of medicine, but medical schools, in general, assign little value to it or to teaching the appropriate skills. We should focus attention on the fundamental importance of communication to the effective practice of medicine through inclusion of specific programs on the subject throughout the medical school curriculum.

Mary Anne C. Johnston

TANA A. GRADY-WELIKY
CYNTHIA N. KETTYLE
EDWARD M. HUNDERT

The Mentor-Mentee Relationship in Medical Education

A New Analysis

In this chapter, we address the professional and personal components of the mentoring relationship in medical education. We begin with a brief review of the literature, which introduces the concept of the mentoring relationship and its critical role in medical student and young physician development. Next we highlight current challenges and opportunities in mentoring relationships and propose two new conceptual matrices for better understanding both professional and personal development within the mentor-mentee dyad. Case examples illustrate the various professional and personal developmental paths described in the two matrices. We conclude by highlighting the specific challenges facing both mentors and mentees in today's changing environment, and by proposing recommendations for growth and improvement in these areas.

Mentoring relationships are fundamental elements of the personal and professional development of physicians, scientists, lawyers, and other professionals. The term *mentor* was introduced in Homer's *Odyssey*, when Telemachus, son of Odysseus, needed someone to help guide him during his father's extended absence. Athena, the goddess of wisdom, disguised herself as Mentor, a visiting male friend of Odysseus, who assisted with Telemachus's growth and development. The relationship between Mentor and Telemachus was comprised of *validating, yet challenging, support*, which helped to foster Telemachus's development from child to adolescent to adult. This type of mentoring relationship has been critical, we believe, in fostering the development of medical students into physicians.

A successful mentoring relationship incorporates both personal and professional development. Faculty members need to pay attention to both components in order to fulfill their half of the mentoring contract. Both mentor and mentee must be willing to understand similarities and differences in their backgrounds and in their career goals and objectives. Faculty members are more effective mentors when they have a comprehensive understanding of medical education innovations, such as enhanced community-based experiences and community service opportunities, and are open to exploring all aspects of medical students' backgrounds in an effort to understand the role these factors may play in their ultimate career goals.

Mentors need to start with a basic assessment of the mentee's level of personal maturity and psychological development. This type of understanding is essential for the mentor to predict and/or to manage how the student will need to develop or enhance coping skills for the stresses of medical school. If a student has endured life circumstances that have prevented a "normal" development, the mentor's understanding of these issues can help guide the student. Such developmental circumstances, which may be different from the mentor's own life experiences, may have contributed to the student's selection of a medical career and may further influence his or her ultimate direction in medicine.

Medical students, as mentees, also bring needs, attitudes, and behaviors to the mentoring relationship that may influence the ability of the mentor to perform his or her function effectively. In general, medical students are intelligent, talented, and energetic people. Some students bring a lifelong dream of providing direct clinical care to patients when they enter medical school. Others are primarily interested in the basic sciences and wish to pursue a career in biomedical research. The majority of students, however, do not have a genuine sense of their particular goals within medicine. Career choice often then becomes a major task for a mentoring "contract."

Personality styles among medical students, which can be quite varied, influence the individual student's interpersonal skills and other behaviors, which in turn influence their "mentorability." For example, students who are extremely inflexible will have difficulty engaging in relationships not only with peers and patients, but also with potential mentors. Central to the mentoring relationship, therefore, are the mentor's ability to recognize such characteristics and his or her willingness to work through them in helping the student define what he/she needs to change and improve.

The significant role of mentors in undergraduate medical education has been described in several studies. Flach and colleagues (1982) developed a faculty mentor program and found strong endorsement of the program by students and faculty, wherein faculty mentors were rated highest as "role models" by students. Igartua (1997) stressed the importance of mentoring as "a faculty priority," noting that "staff who take on the responsibility of guiding students through their training must be recognized for their important contribution to medical edu-

Tana A. Grady-Weliky, Cynthia N. Kettyle, and Edward M. Hundert

cation" (p. 3). This report also found that similarities between mentor and student (same gender and similar career interests) might foster the relationship and influence the personal component of the mentor-mentee dyad. Still, the impact of such similarities on students' ultimate professional development is less clear. For example, midlevel and senior women faculty members have anecdotally noted the positive influence that male mentors have had on their professional development during medical school and residency.

Reuler and Nardone (1994) examined the difference between role models and mentors in medical education. They describe the mentoring relationship as "more continuous and complex than that of a role model" (p. 335), in that role models typically teach by example and subsequently shape professional identity through inspiration. This is different from the notion of a mentor who serves as an intellectual guide and facilitator of growth and change in the mentee. They further urge medical educators to address the diverse medical student body with a more representative faculty who could serve as role models, asserting that "the predominance of white men on the faculty of many medical schools may contribute to the stress that many women or minority students and residents feel" (p. 336). In the Flach study (1982), age and gender, as well as medical specialty of the mentor, did indeed have an effect on the student-mentor relationship.

Studies of junior faculty development have also examined the influence of gender on the quality of mentoring relationships. In their examination of women's career development in internal medicine, Fried and colleagues (1996) found that the quality of mentoring differed by gender of the mentor and junior faculty mentee. While both men and women junior faculty equally reported having mentors, there were significant differences in the likelihood of mentors facilitating the junior faculty members' participation in conferences and invited manuscripts. Male junior faculty members were more likely to have mentors who promoted their participation in these activities, whereas female junior faculty members were more likely to have mentors who used their work to advance their own careers rather than mentees' careers. Women were also more likely to identify difficulty in the mentoring relationship when the mentor and mentee were different genders compared to same-sex mentoring dyads. Yet Palepu and colleagues (1998) found that 80 percent of the women faculty and 86 percent of the minority faculty surveyed did not believe it was important to have a mentor of the same gender or race, respectively. This finding would corroborate anecdotal reports of women faculty members who have not reported significant problems with male mentors with regard to professional development.

In retrospect, the early Greek notion of the mentoring relationship is rather straightforward and simple, particularly in light of the presumed similarities in gender and culture between Telemachus and Mentor. The rapidly changing demographics of medical students, in combination with the paradigm shifts in health care delivery in our current academic medicine environment, create new challenges to the mentoring concept. As mentoring medical educators, we must examine the impact of a heterogeneous student body in a largely homogeneous academic medicine environment. Mentors will need to continue to nurture, support, and educate students. However, they may be faced with the challenges of students who have different backgrounds and who may bring innovative ideas regarding medical careers and professional development to the mentoring relationship. With this in mind, the new mentoring tasks will include enhanced sensitivity and openness to students with different backgrounds and professional goals, and the ability to relate to and respect this diversity of cultures and interests.

A faculty development process to enhance the mentoring skills of senior faculty is central to effecting change and improving the usefulness of mentoring relationships. To this end, Wright and colleagues (1998) suggest that faculty can be taught to become outstanding mentors through the identification and appreciation of mentee differences. Another opportunity for an improved mentor-mentee relationship lies in the use of closer linkages between academic health centers and community-based health care settings. Several medical schools have incorporated partnerships with health-care- and non–health-care-related community service organizations into the undergraduate curriculum, thereby enhancing, in one instance, the cross-cultural training of medical students (Nora, Daugherty, Mattis-Peterson, Stevenson, & Goodman, 1994).

In this chapter, we will offer a conceptual matrix for approaching these issues, using cases to demonstrate the potential impact of traditional mentors on nontraditional students who have backgrounds and/or goals similar to or different from the mentor. Also included in the matrix are examples of how traditional mentors might better understand the traditional student with nontraditional career goals. In addition, we review the specific challenges and opportunities facing medical educators, mentors, and students in today's medical education environment.

Traditional and Nontraditional Backgrounds and Career Goals: Challenges to Mentoring Professional Development

In a world that has (and needs) increasing numbers of medical students from nontraditional backgrounds — and where many students from either traditional or nontraditional backgrounds may have an interest in pursuing non-

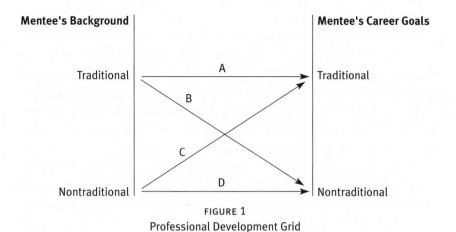

Mentee's Background

Traditional

Nontraditional

Mentee's Career Goals

Traditional

Nontraditional

A

B

C

D

FIGURE 1
Professional Development Grid

traditional careers — the mentoring paradigm given us by the *Odyssey* is too simple. As we saw above, Telemachus wants and needs to grow up to be like his father; if his father is gone, his father's friend Mentor takes over the job with most of the same attributes and values that would have been provided by the father. In the Professional Development Grid shown in figure 1, this situation is represented by arrow A, indicating the traditional model of mentoring. In the story, Mentor is there to reinforce the values that Telemachus should hold, and to introduce him into the right circles to nurture his "success" in the dominant culture. Although there are challenges in the traditional mentor-mentee dyad related to personality characteristics on either side of the equation, the framework and mentoring "contract" remain relatively clear.

Things become more complicated as we look at the other three potential paths in the Professional Development Grid (fig. 1). In arrow B we are faced with a student from a traditional background who desires a nontraditional outcome, defined in terms relevant to the local culture. Here we start with a traditional student, say, a white male from an upper-middle-class background with a physician parent. But this student wants to get training in acupuncture and massage therapy parallel with his training in internal medicine. Another such student might want to practice as the sole physician on an island or in a remote area, but is studying at an institution where everyone around him is steering (and being steered) toward academic medicine. Another is pursuing a career in family medicine in a medical center that does not even have such a department. One could even put into the same category the mentoring of students choosing careers not traditional for their gender, such as female students with an interest in surgery or, now, male students with an interest in obstetrics and gynecology.

Obviously, these students and their needs challenge the dominant paradigm and raise issues about the school's stated mission. Here the mentees often can act as change agents, broadening the de facto mission of the school. Moreover, the emerging shift to community-based medicine with a population perspective will challenge mentors to broaden their view on the role of community experiences and their impact on the professional development of students. The Pew Health Professions Committee (1994) developed a set of core competencies for physicians in 2005, including care for the community's health, practice prevention, and participation in racially and culturally diverse society. O'Neil and Seifer (1995) note that "opportunities for training beyond the walls of the traditional academic medical center will help physicians-in-training to acquire the competencies demanded by a reformed health care system and its consumers" (p. S42). As increasing numbers of medical student participate in community and other educational activities beyond the medical school classroom, mentors will be challenged by students to grow beyond narrow visions of the goals of medical education. This growth will facilitate the development of a more effective mentor-mentee relationship, particularly along the path of the traditional student with nontraditional career goals.

Consider, however, the following. We have all probably been faced with a female student who has always been a highly achievement-oriented, driven individual and who appears to be choosing surgery in no small part because it is the most challenging career she can contemplate. How does one mentor such a student if one truly believes that pathological levels of the usual "achievement neurosis" are actually leading a student down a career path of great personal dissatisfaction? In at least five such cases from our collective experience, we can report that personal suffering was almost inevitable when mentors supported without challenge these students' choice of surgery. In all five cases, despite a dazzling residency record and over the protests of each of the training directors, each student ended up abandoning her choice in midresidency, with mentors and, indeed, friends, quietly shaking their heads, thinking "I *should have* told you so." Of course, there are even more examples in the other direction, where a student legitimately wants to carve out a unique career path for all the right reasons and is pressured to conform by mentors and friends alike, again leading to a dissatisfying career, always wishing she had chosen an alternative career path. These cases highlight the need for a deep level of trust on both sides of the relationship, so that difficult and delicate questions can be posed and considered by both parties.

The issues and potential biases represented in arrow C on the Professional

Tana A. Grady-Weliky, Cynthia N. Kettyle, and Edward M. Hundert

Development Grid are no less complex. The very existence of more nontraditional applicants and matriculants in medical school classes has become a focus of considerable national attention, since this group includes underrepresented minorities caught in the affirmative action debate. But this group also includes many older students who present unique mentoring challenges, such as a former corporate CEO or school principal now placed in the infantilizing role of a first-year medical student. It also includes students from other stigmatized groups — gay and lesbian students, certain foreign nationals, or even students from traditional backgrounds who simply act or look different from most of their classmates. We have seen these issues arise with everything from a severely obese student to a student with body piercing to male students with long hair to female students sporting crewcuts.

Students in this category who want to follow arrow C to a traditional career are often treated by mentors in the same way as students traveling along arrow A. Many mentors will put them in this category, simply "reinforce" traditional values, and introduce them into the standard power groups. But below the surface it makes no sense to talk about "reinforcing" values for people whose background or identity may include a different set of values.

Indeed, one could view arrow C as an arrow of bias, turning students away from their own values and beliefs to those serving the dominant culture. A major challenge presented to mentors here is whether they can or even should question the student's desire to achieve a more traditional outcome. Again, one can step into a nightmare if a Hispanic student from a poor family wants to become a subspecialist in an affluent suburb: what role should a mentor play in helping that student understand this desire? Even to raise the question steps onto a slope where one could argue that, if the same questions were not asked of students traveling along arrow A, there must be an implicit assumption that this student was admitted to medical school for the express purpose of returning him to his community to care for "his people." Even if the decision is made to support without challenge the desired outcome, this student will often need a lot more practical advice to help him succeed and to cope with the biases of others he will meet along the way.

When we come at last to arrow D of the grid, we can begin to question how mainstream (traditional) mentors can really be of any help. Perhaps the most complicated of all combinations is the student of one nontraditional category who seeks to end up in a nontraditional place. The development of nontraditional mentors for these students is not limited to increasing numbers of faculty from nontraditional or underrepresented minority backgrounds within academic medical centers. We also need to look to other, community-based locations as potential sites where mentoring can take place. With this in mind, medical educators should continue to foster partnerships with the community in an effort to enhance the mentorship of our students.

Normal and Pathological Personal Development: Challenges to Mentoring Personal Growth

It must be true that Mentor was indeed Athena, the goddess of wisdom, because we are told that what Mentor offered to Telemachus to foster his growth and development was *validating, yet challenging, support*. Mentor was very wise indeed to understand that a delicate balance of challenge and validation is necessary.

The modern medical student would her- or himself be a challenge to Mentor. Medical education is a profound stimulus for growth and change. As medical educators know only too well, some students thrive on the personal and professional challenge, while others are overwhelmed by some aspects of the experience. Admissions committees use every means at their disposal to evaluate the strengths of applicants and to assess their developmental level and capacity to grow, but the science of applicant selection is far from exact.

In addition to the large group of students whose personal development has been normal and will continue to be so throughout the challenges of medical training, medical school classes also contain some students who display significant psychopathology, and some who will develop problems as they encounter challenges. The possible paths are summarized in the Personal Development Grid (fig. 2).

We can infer from *The Odyssey* that attention to the personal development of the mentee falls under the purview of the mentor. This statement warrants particular emphasis, as it is often this responsibility which receives the least conscious attention. Possible reasons for this neglect include concern about the political correctness of scrutinizing or influencing the personal life of the mentee; uncertainty about how to assess developmental issues and what to do with the data obtained; and difficulties in the mentor's own personal growth and development that make the task threatening or impossible.

It is also true, however, that a mentor's assessment of the personal development of his/her mentee may be largely intuitive and may actively inform many aspects of the interactions. This would be most likely in the case described by arrow 1 in the Personal Development Grid.

Tana A. Grady-Weliky, Cynthia N. Kettyle, and Edward M. Hundert

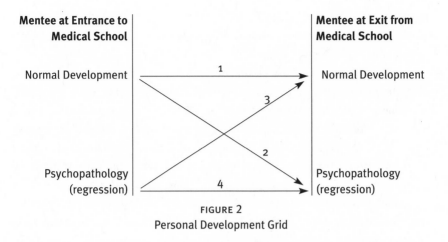

FIGURE 2
Personal Development Grid

The scenarios scripted by arrows 2, 3, and 4 on the grid are those which pose the greatest challenge to the mentor, but also the most compelling reasons for the role to exist. Take the case of a psychologically healthy student who loses ground developmentally as he or she becomes immersed in the rigors of medical school. An example is provided by a young woman from an economically disadvantaged family in an isolated rural area of the Midwest who left home for the first time at age sixteen to attend a small liberal arts college on the East Coast. Although young for her age in some ways, and younger chronologically than her peers, she worked very hard in her academic pursuits, majoring in biophysics, and went directly to medical school after college. She met the challenge of the basic sciences in the first-year curriculum with ease. She also made significant strides in areas of personal development. She became more interested in and trusting of friends, more outgoing socially, and more confident and assertive in peer-group activities. During her second year, however, a pattern consistent with arrow 2 was observed. The clinical opportunities introduced during that year were difficult for her, and she avoided interactions with real patients as much as possible. As courses and tutorials became less structured, her grades dropped. Her social activities became more and more constricted. By the end of her second year she experienced a major depressive episode, resulting in a medical leave of absence.

Although her relationship with her mentor was affected by the changes described, it was the mentor's appreciation of the signs and symptoms of growth, then regression, and finally clear-cut psychopathology that proved most helpful in the nurture, support, and education of this young woman. Her mentor was able to advocate (an important term which we explain below) on her behalf with faculty and administration. Most important, the mentor supported her ultimate decision to move away from medicine and toward a career which she found less threatening and more fulfilling.

In light of the Personal Development Grid, it is interesting to reconsider the cases discussed in the previous section in which five students with "pathological achievement neurosis" all selected the most challenging career (surgery), only to abandon this path in midresidency. Had mentors successfully addressed issues of personal growth, perhaps these individuals could have been steered along arrow 3 on the Personal Development Grid. While there are many paths to an "achievement neurosis," it is often the result of psychological defense mechanisms that protect the individual from awareness of some vulnerability, fear, or inadequacy. Such individuals often exhibit attitudes of exaggerated self-confidence, certainty, and assertiveness. They often appear unidimensional in their focus and have developed certain areas of their life to the detriment of other areas, for which they show disdain. They may appear to others as arrogant and controlling, and yet have no insight into how they are seen. The underlying psychopathology may be serious and pervasive or more circumscribed, and it may be the product of a particular stress that medical training provokes in the individual. In either case, without some intervention, a student may choose his/her career poorly, based on a defensive distortion of who the student really is, and what he or she really wants. Those mentors who shook their heads, thinking, "I *should have* told you so," not only missed an important window of opportunity, but also revealed their naiveté regarding personal development. Before intervention, the psychopathology or developmental pitfalls must first be recognized, and a plan formulated. The psychologically vulnerable medical student can then move from a position of partial compromise to one in which new growth and development occur and are integrated into the personality.

Most discouraging, perhaps, is arrow 4 on the grid, which represents the student who suffers from significant personal limitations from matriculation through graduation. Those limitations may shift, get better with maturing development, or get worse if the challenges of the medical school years are not met with much-needed personal growth. Several examples come to mind of students whose names appeared with regularity on the Promotions Board Committee's meeting agenda. The limitations may appear in academic performance or in concerns regarding character, behavior, socialization, or professionalism.

A student whose difficulties spanned several of these areas illustrates this path — a young woman whose mentor would say, "It's always something!" Early in the first year she had trouble disciplining herself to keep up with daily and weekly assignments. There were too many things to do. Faculty feedback sug-

Tana A. Grady-Weliky, Cynthia N. Kettyle, and Edward M. Hundert

gested she was not prepared for classes or tests. Her grades were poor. Mild symptoms of depression appeared. She fell further behind in her work and could not follow through on remedial plans carefully negotiated with her by faculty members. She was distracted by breakups with boyfriends, quarrels with her parents, and clashes with her roommate. She moved out of the dorm. She couldn't get along with a new landlord who accused her of stealing. The story goes on, but it doesn't change very much. What is a mentor to do?

The mentor's experience was frustrating and time consuming. As is the case at all levels of the medical profession, the unmentorable student or colleague consumes a disproportionate share of resources, and often very little progress is made. It is fair to say that this student entered medical school with significant character pathology. The mentor's arsenal of support and the mission to nurture and educate were powerless in the face of a developmental arrest.

A discussion of the skills and techniques necessary for successful mentoring of personal and professional development can facilitate the experience. In both areas a mentoring "contract" is necessary. Some explicit understanding of the purposes and goals, as well as the limitations, of the relationship must be shared by mentor and mentee. The parameters of the relationship should be clarified, including the availability of the mentor, and the purpose and format of meetings.

Not every mentor needs psychiatric training, but some appreciation of certain psychological phenomena is crucial in the mentor's approach to the mentee. The psychiatrist's concept of *transference* is most important for any mentor to understand. Attitudes, impulses, feelings, and fantasies from significant early relationships (especially parents) are likely to be repeated unconsciously in the mentor-mentee relationship. Transference often explains an emotional valence in the relationship which may or may not be appropriate. Other signs of transference might be an exaggerated response or inappropriate set of assumptions or expectations. Transference is not necessarily good or bad, useful or not, in a mentoring situation, but it is important to recognize its contribution to the relationship.

Equally important in mentoring is an awareness of psychological defense mechanisms. Medical school is an undertaking that promises to provide significant stress throughout. In order for growth to occur in both personal and professional domains, stress must be kept at a tolerable level. Since defense mechanisms distort reality, the conscious presentation of thought or emotions may be quite different from what is really going on for the student. The cases discussed in the professional development section of this chapter highlight this point. The choice of those five students, selecting what they considered to be the hardest specialty, may reflect a defensive distortion, resulting in a counterphobic career plan. In fact, all career paths illustrated in the Professional Development Grid (fig. 1, arrows A, B, C, and D) can be heavily influenced by defense, and the astute mentor must factor this into his/her approach.

Mentoring, by definition, is a process that occurs over time. It is important to recognize from the outset that a successful mentoring relationship will be one that deepens and grows. An element that can be seen as the core of the relationship between mentor and mentee is their alliance. Analogous as it is to the concept of a therapeutic alliance in the doctor-patient relationship, we might call it the "mentoring alliance." Simply put, it refers to the healthy and mature aspects of *both* mentor and mentee who together form an alliance centered around the task of furthering the personal and professional development of the mentee. It requires some basic trust to get off the ground, and it must be monitored as the relationship progresses. Serious negative feelings or reactions within the dyad can rupture the mentoring alliance and preclude further work. Institutional provisions should be in place to deal with this possibility.

The concept of advocacy logically follows a discussion of the mentoring alliance. It is our belief that the mentor is in a unique position to serve as an advocate for the mentee, but only if advocacy is consistent with the mentor's charge to "support, nurture, and educate" the mentee. All too often, advocacy is seen as getting the student out of trouble of some kind or minimizing the severity of disciplinary actions. Needless to say, such interventions may actually interfere with more effective measures. A resilient mentoring alliance is essential in these difficult situations. The case of the young woman who, with the support of her mentor, left medical school for another successful career is a reminder that the traditional assumptions of both arrow 1 and arrow A are not always relevant: both mentor and mentee saw her decision to leave medicine gracefully as proof of the success of the mentoring alliance.

Finally, how does one say goodbye? Psychoanalysts would remind us that the termination of a therapeutic relationship is a stimulus for growth. Ideally, when a junior person has been supported, challenged, and helped by a senior person, there has been a transmission of values, skills, attitudes, and behaviors that becomes part of the identity of the trainee. Termination of the mentoring relationship may solidify this identification. In the medical community, where mentees often become colleagues of their mentors, perhaps even within the same institution, termination of the mentoring relationship and transition to a collegial one is the final challenge, a developmental milestone for both mentor and mentee alike.

In this chapter, we have presented some of the complexities of the mentoring relationship. Important factors which contribute to the success or failure

Tana A. Grady-Weliky, Cynthia N. Kettyle, and Edward M. Hundert

of the process include the receptivity of the mentee, the expertise of the mentor, the openness of the mentor to acknowledging the role of educational experiences in community-based and other innovative settings, and the appropriateness of the match between mentor and mentee. We have proposed two matrices to help focus thinking about that relationship, one with respect to professional development and the other with respect to personal development. Our conclusions, based on hundreds of observations of mentoring, good and bad, could be translated into a number of recommendations for action. We might group these recommendations into three categories, as discussed separately below: (1) selection issues for mentors and mentees; (2) development programs to enhance both the mentee receptor and the mentor substrate; and (3) programs to nurture and support mentoring over time.

––––––––

All of the references cited above on the mentoring relationship include some observations about the selection of mentors who can support junior colleagues and act as role models for the best attributes of physicians. The very best mentors are often readily identified by generations of students and residents who have connected with this small group of remarkable faculty over the years. Selecting mentors who are "merely" very good is trickier. As noted above, a good mentor must possess a combination of important qualities, both interpersonal and intellectual. It is important to select mentors who will give this important activity the time and attention it deserves. It is also important not to select just anyone who says she/he has the time to give, since some faculty members have time available because they are not succeeding in other areas of their careers!

Additionally, the importance of diversity and the need for mentors from nontraditional and underrepresented minority backgrounds make a strong case for pipeline programs to produce mentors for the next generation, who will need a more diverse group of mentors than is currently available. Mentors need to have enthusiasm for the assignment, satisfaction with their own professional accomplishments, openness to the thoughts, feelings, and opinions of others, psychological sophistication, and personal maturity. Most of all, mentors should be selected because they are the sort of people who truly get joy from nurturing and celebrating the achievement of others, remaining in the background to support but not overshadow their mentee's successes. Indeed, the best mentors probably do this, directly or indirectly, as a result of an identification with and in gratitude to the mentors who did the same for them.

Much less attention has been paid to the selection of mentorable mentees. Since mentoring is so central to professional development, we believe that interviewers for medical school admissions should try to assess the "mentee receptor" of applicants. This could be done in a direct way, asking applicants about people who have been influential in the applicant's thinking about career choices. What if a student responds that he or she "never got to know any one faculty member all that well in that way"? While the interviewer may diagnose a deprived academic environment, the interviewer may also wonder whether this suggests a defective mentee receptor. In such cases, the matter should be pursued further before the usual reliance on MCATS and GPAs misses the most important admissions diagnosis. On the other hand, it is less important that applicants mention faculty members, so long as they mention *some* individual — grandparent, friend of the family, or any person — an attachment to whom furthered personal growth.

The medical school admission process selects people who are good at reading what the environment expects of them — and then meeting these expectations. The implication, of course, is that, since we know students are so expectation-sensitive, we are most likely to have an impact upon the mentor-mentee interaction if we work more on improving the mentoring environment.

––––––––

As with selection, there has been more attention paid to programs that might develop mentors than to those focused on the development of mentees. Such mentor-development programs need to include some basics in the development of young adults. Faculty need support on fostering a mentoring contract that includes both support and challenge. They need support in establishing "mentoring alliances" over time, with personal help for them from a mentor's Mentor when challenging situations arise.

We believe that inattention to the personal development side of mentoring has led to many missed opportunities; the focus of the relationship may become entirely career-oriented, in part because of the mentor's discomfort at getting involved in other complex issues. Since an absence of appreciation for developmental psychological factors can itself thwart efforts to support career development, the need for some basic training in young adult development represents another recommendation that grows out of the perspective painted here, since the two grids proposed in this chapter are completely intertwined.

Equally important, we believe that programs must be developed to help mentees develop their own mentee receptors, their receptivity to mentoring. From the first week of medical school, students can be taught about the need for mentoring, the tasks of mentoring, and the best ways to strengthen the mentoring relationship. This amounts to a curriculum of education about mentoring for both mentors and mentees. Many schools are currently trying to revise their advising systems, and at least two schools have changed the structure of the office of student affairs to create a cohort of "advisory deans" who can take on the student affairs role for a small group of students. At the University of Rochester and at Duke, each advisory dean gets to know his or her cohort of students over the four years, to help develop their "mentorability" and also to help them create a network with other faculty to enhance the likelihood of connecting with a faculty mentor in their career interest.

Ultimately what is needed is the support of a *culture of mentoring*. The academic medical culture has recently been described in terms of the "informal" or "hidden" curriculum (Bickel, 1996; Hafferty, 1998; Hundert, Bickel, & Douglas-Steele, 1996). Every school should have formal and highly public awards for mentoring, programs to mentor the mentors, and support for mentors over time. Does a mentor who is in a difficult mentoring relationship have a senior person to whom he or she can go for support in terminating the relationship in a positive way? Is there a routine procedure to monitor the program and effect changes when indicated? Simple assignment of mentors may not work, since the mentor and mentee need a task on which to work together to become junior and senior colleagues, rather than just "friends." Schools can develop guidelines and programs to make pairing assignments more carefully and to sustain them over time, collecting and interpreting data that will facilitate more-successful future assignments. Schools must also recognize that mentors change over time. Sometimes a junior faculty member who wants and perhaps needs to be more focused on his or her own career development might become a highly valued mentor once he/she feels freer to focus on nurturing the success of others. In this sense, the same life-cycle perspective we take with mentees must be taken equally with mentors.

To our knowledge, however, no medical school has yet taken the bold step of formalizing criteria for mentoring in the promotions process. But if this is as important as most people believe, perhaps there is no excuse for failing to do so. As promotions committees count first authorships in major journals toward full professorships, perhaps the time has come to require a certain number of *last* authorships, with mentees as first authors, before promotion to full professor. If these and other guidelines document in the mentor's CV or dossier the extent to which that mentor promoted his or her mentee's career, *as criteria for promotion*, this may well do more than any other awards program to nurture a culture of mentoring that would support both mentees and mentors.

NORMA E. WAGONER

From Identity Purgatory to Professionalism

Considerations along the Medical Education Continuum

Although medical educators fully realize that the medical school environment serves in many ways as an incubator of professionalism, rarely do we examine its strengths and weaknesses relative to this purpose (Hafferty, 1998). If we use public satisfaction with physicians as a gauge, we have much room to improve. Students come to medical school with high ideals and expectations, eager to adopt the standards of their chosen profession, but somewhere along the line many lose resolve.

While they seek a clear set of ethical standards, they encounter instead a multitude of vague, abstract definitions of what it means to be a professional. As they progress, many students begin to doubt themselves and enter into an identity purgatory that further jeopardizes their ability to acquire the professional values we hope to instill. As educators, we need to take definitive steps to alter the traditional model of medical education in order to more effectively inculcate in our students the crucial elements of professionalism: altruism, accountability, excellence, duty to service, honor, integrity, and respect for others (ABIM, 1999).

In this chapter, I discuss some of the social and cultural elements in medical education that contribute to students' conflicts about professionalism. Second, I look at the formal curriculum, including typical admissions procedures, and the steps that have been taken at the Pritzker School of Medicine to address the specific challenges posed by each medical school year. Last, I turn to the informal curriculum, including mentoring programs, to student activism in the community, and to the need for evaluation of both student progress and that of medical schools in the new managed care environment.

In my twenty-five years as a dean of students and professor of anatomy, I have heard many students express concerns about becoming true professionals. Having closely examined their own moral and ethical values, perhaps for the first time in their lives, they wonder how they will reach the elusive goal of being a professional. How will they acquire the necessary principles? Is professionalism something extra they must learn in addition to biomedical knowledge and skills, or will this quality just come to them? As students grapple with these questions, their definitions of themselves within the context of medicine begin to blur. What is it we do as educators to inflict this identity purgatory on so many students? Is it a necessary phase in professional development, or can we somehow prevent such conflicts from occurring?

Some historical perspective on these questions is in order. During the first half of my years in the medical school environment, educators often discussed the subject of professionalism. Not until the late 1970s and early 1980s did sociologists suggest that the two-hundred-year-old work ethic had begun to erode in the United States. During that period Daniel Yankelovich (1981) explored how this shift in society's pluralistic values was changing today's young people. He contended that the traditional ethic of delayed gratification and unremitting toil had been replaced by one that denies the individual nothing. Indeed, today's medical students value personal freedom even more than did those in the 1980s, often to the extent that they view each new commitment as a threat to their autonomy. While there is nothing intrinsically wrong with this attitude, it does conflict with the values of most senior faculty members, who were brought up under the old work ethic.

A second schism of values derives from the fact that students now come from many different cultures and backgrounds, instilled with the moral precepts integral to their upbringing. This diversity has two important implications. First, what many consider an obvious ethical indiscretion may be seen by students from other cultures as perfectly acceptable behavior. For instance, a basic-science faculty member at Pritzker told me that, out of curiosity, she had asked three postdoctoral fellows from different countries what they would do if they witnessed a student cheating. The first one responded, "It wouldn't bother me"; the second one said, "Everybody cheats; if you don't, you are the loser"; and the third one remarked, "I would just hope that he wasn't dumb enough to get caught." Unfortunately, many faculty members still teach as if all students share a common moral foundation. Given obvious diversities, we need to consider what remedial steps we could take to help our faculty and staff better relate to students.

A third area of dysfunction relates to the intense competition to gain entrance to medical school. Most students spend their premedical school years focused exclusively on attaining the high academic ratings the schools require. A high proportion of students choose not to participate in sports, music, or any other extracurricular activity that would detract from their academic concentration.

This single-minded focus limits students' abilities to develop resourcefulness and coping skills. They thrive on perfection and rarely experience failure within the structured safety of academia; the fear of failing becomes the modus operandi of their lives. As a result, some of these highly achieving students suffer substantial difficulties in the unstructured environment of medical school.

I believe that in addition to the guidance and support inherent in a humanistic environment, we can further ensure that our students acquire the principles of humanism through a continuum of experiences that reinforce the importance of professional values. Along a planned continuum, we could incorporate formal curricular offerings, curricular enhancement programs, events, and ceremonies that emphasize and reward professional behavior. Also, to whatever extent possible, we should provide positive learning experiences within the informal curriculum. By regularly monitoring and evaluating our progress, we can be assured of educating more competent and caring physicians. To be certain, despite our utmost efforts, students will inevitably face moral dilemmas and negative ordeals within the informal curriculum. It is our responsibility as medical educators to prepare students ahead of time with the guidance and understanding necessary to deal with these dilemmas in a way that promotes, rather than detracts from, their professional growth and socialization.

The Formal Curriculum: Institutional Policies and the Curriculum

As Reiser notes in part 1 of this book, our mission statements and institutional policies, whether intentionally or not, make clear declarations about professionalism. Some schools have also developed codes of conduct, which, unfortunately, often focus on what constitutes unacceptable, rather than meritorious, behavior. To be sure, a code of conduct may protect the school by outlining standards and procedures dealing with incompetent or unethical students. But an important opportunity is lost if codes do not also make an affirmative statement about what the institution values.

———

It can scarcely be denied that students have developed their standards of ethics and key character traits by the time they enter medical school. Seymour Glick observed that "medical training can disillusion and render cynical even some quite decent students, but rarely can it convert a basically self-centered and egotistic person into a humanitarian" (1981, p. 1038). Medical educators therefore assume an obligation to select candidates who already possess sound ethical values. Yet medical schools continue to admit candidates who lack commitment, proper motives, appropriate personalities, or adequate communication and social skills. This occurs primarily because admissions committees continue to base their selection of students on test scores and grade point averages (Oransky & Savitz, 1998). Our admissions process must identify individuals who will not only succeed as students, but who also have both the practical and altruistic qualities necessary to care for patients in the evolving constraints and opportunities of this new century.

In June of 1998, the Arnold P. Gold Foundation organized and supported a conference titled "Challenging the Barriers to Sustaining Humanism in Medicine: Selecting Humanistic Candidates for Medical School." While none of the following recommendations are new, they deserve re-statement: (1) devise an evaluation instrument for admissions committees that assesses competency and humanism; (2) formally train committee members to recognize ethical and moral characteristics; (3) select humanistic committee members, such as religious and community leaders and schoolteachers; (4) identify resources that allow for at least two interviews per applicant; and (5) make certain that committees evaluate applicants fairly (Arnold P. Gold Foundation, 1998).

If the applicant pool declines precipitously, medical schools will be faced with even more difficult choices. Will we reduce class sizes? Must we populate the ranks with those who don't measure up to the desired humanistic standards? By its nature a heroic profession, the practice of medicine should focus first and foremost on service to others and on meeting public health goals.

———

Charged with lofty standards and idealistic expectations, entering students assume that once accepted they will be treated consistently with respect, honesty, and tolerance. They are shocked when they witness physicians, staff, and peers acting without integrity. At a seminar for sophomore students on professionalism, we asked them to define what they considered unprofessional behavior among faculty. Two descriptions prevailed: dehumanization of students, colleagues, patients, and others by showing lack of respect, breach of confidentiality, displays of intolerance, or dishonesty; and insensitivities based on gender, ethnicity, or cultural beliefs, particularly involving racist or sexist remarks.

Competition also proves extremely detrimental to students' morale and progress by precluding their ability to attend to physical and emotional needs, spend time with friends and family, and participate in community or other extracurricular activities. Wear (1997) succinctly sums up the problem of competition: "The very structure of medical training promotes such fact grubbing and hyper-competitiveness that the goals of caring for anything other than grades and class rank are often lost in the medical school scramble. In such an academic environment, the hyper-competitiveness of the students parallels and is fed by the hyper-competitiveness of the faculty" (p. 1056). At Pritzker we use a pass-fail system, which has helped reduce competition among students. Schools unable to change their grading systems should consider instituting programmatic efforts that foster cooperation, such as group projects in which students receive a common evaluation. Group projects enable students to put aside their competitive preoccupation, reduce their feelings of isolation, and become more effective team members.

In addition to the above-mentioned hindrances, students encounter other less apparent obstacles. In a 1997 conference on humanism in medicine, students, residents, deans, and educators identified many of these barriers, including two that are particularly germane here: lack of open communication with classmates, and the pessimistic attitude of older students (Arnold P. Gold Foundation, 1997). All of these impediments diminish students' confidence and make them doubt their abilities to become professionals.

In light of these hindrances, our first goal should be to impart *clear expectations* regarding professional behavior. Students come from a variety of backgrounds and cultures, and even the most altruistic can become confused about professionalism. Meaningful ethics teaching infused throughout the entire curriculum would appear crucial (Hundert, 1996). Yet we occasionally receive feedback from students indicating that they couldn't relate to what they learned in ethics classes, that they simply heard the standard commentary about abortion, euthanasia, informed consent, fetal tissue, and so on. From listening to students, I have concluded (as have others before me) that, in order to be truly helpful, ethics courses must aid students in assessing and clarifying their own values (Bickel, 1987, 1996; Christakis & Feudtner, 1993; Hafferty, 1998; Hafferty & Franks, 1994). At the same time, the course content should contain basic ethical guidelines on caring for patients, including the significance of patient preference and quality-of-life issues. Such a foundation would furnish a guide to students during medical school and throughout their careers.

In addition to improving our ethics classes, we should encourage and evaluate faculty on their demonstrations of integrity, compassion, and other humanistic qualities. As Reiser emphasizes, students working toward self-definition pay close attention to faculty members, and every display of integrity, compassion, and respect that they witness, whether toward patients, staff, or students, sends a strong message about what it means to be a professional.

At Pritzker we offer many milestone ceremonies and events for first- and second-year students. These events not only prove inspirational, they serve other purposes, strengthening ties to those faculty who have proven to be excellent role models, giving students an opportunity to gain leadership and organization abilities, and increasing students' confidence. One of the programs we have instituted is a four-day orientation for incoming freshmen, which our second-year students develop and conduct as a symbolic gift to them. Prior to the orientation, selected sophomores reflect on their own first-year experiences and, based on their findings, devise a program aimed at helping new students overcome anxiety, establish coping mechanisms, be resourceful, and build relationships with those who can give them proper guidance.

In 1989, we instituted a white coat ceremony as part of freshman orientation, to serve as a formal induction into the profession of medicine. Sophomores choose as the speaker a physician who they believe best represents the ideals of humanism. They select another physician to present each first-year student with a white coat, stethoscope, ethics book, and the book *On Doctoring* (Reynolds and Stone, 1995), a gift from the Robert Wood Johnson Foundation to every medical student in the country. In proffering these symbols, each of which also has practical value, we welcome our students into the profession. A faculty member leads the students in a recitation of the modified Hippocratic oath, reinforcing the tenets of professionalism. This ceremony, with an average attendance of five hundred, is highly valued by students, families, and the school. Over the past decade, with the help of the Arnold P. Gold Foundation, more than 108 of the nation's 125 medical schools have adopted this ceremony.

At the beginning of the winter quarter we give our first-year students a booklet entitled "Now Is the Time, Residency Is a Four-Year Process." This booklet, which I wrote based on student questions posed to me during presentations on the residency selection process, follows a question-and-answer format aimed at prompting students to consider career goals and to view choices they make as they relate to future planning. After winter-quarter midterms, the dean of students' office hosts a freshman retreat, organized by sophomores, fifty miles from the campus. The entire freshman class attends, along with fifteen faculty members (and their children), selected by the hosting sophomores, and approximately thirty sophomores, juniors, and seniors. Programmatic components include a stress-management workshop given by a graduate who is a psychiatrist, and a "What's My Type" workshop using the Myers-Briggs instrument and led by a clinical psychologist. These workshops offer students insights into their own behavior as well as that of others. Faculty-led seminars cover subjects selected by first-year students, such as career and family issues, death and dying, challenges to women as physicians and mothers, and the future of medicine. Students have several opportunities on both formal and informal occasions during the retreat to discuss personal, professional, or ethical issues they have encountered during their first five months of medical school.

At the request of a recent sophomore class, we initiated a second-year orientation program to provide an overview of the coming year, including making choices about rotation sequences and preparing for the USMLE Step 1. We furnish second-year students with updated information about the residency selection process and impress upon them the importance of considering career goals in anticipation of this process.

———

Many factors combine to make the third year highly stressful for students. The transition from the structured classroom to an unstructured clinical environment causes consternation for many students. As the year progresses, competition and time limitations add to their turmoil. On the wards, students face a significant dilemma in deciding between "rocking the boat" or "being a team player." As Bickel summarizes, "Seeing that their learning often comes at the expense of patients is emotionally difficult, and pressures to fit in usually guarantee that such worries go unexpressed" (1996, p. 634). Students worry about what will be expected of them in each clerkship, and struggle to interpret their clinical evaluations. Other matters outside the curriculum continue to beg for students' attention, including studying for national boards, making career plans, and applying for residency programs. When moral dilemmas arise, students can scarcely pause to analyze their feelings, assess what they have learned, reflect on their professional growth, or find a role model with whom to discuss their problems.

In order to ameliorate and counteract these stresses, at Pritzker we conduct a third-year orientation and ceremony, during which we provide students with details about upcoming clerkships and help them celebrate their transition to their most important year in becoming professionals. The Arnold P. Gold Foundation has provided support for the ceremony, and Pritzker has served as one of five pilot schools for the program. Each year, prior to the ceremony, third-year students vote on six outstanding residents whom they wish to honor as humanistic teachers and role models. One year a chief resident and graduate of the school presented students with a list of "commonsense tips on succeeding

Norma E. Wagoner

in third year." Ten residents led small-group discussions of the "one hundred greatest student fears." One of the graduates of the medical school presented her story as a patient, since her illness brought her to the intensive care unit a number of times in her senior year. As a prelude to a final faculty-led discussion, the students watched a video that depicted the roles of attending, resident, and student in the palliative care of a dying patient. We closed the formal presentations by having a practicing physician review the modified Hippocratic oath in terms of what it meant at this stage of a professional life. Students were given journals, and we impressed upon them the importance of taking time during their third year to write about and reflect on pivotal events that occur, particularly those that challenge their beliefs and values. In the most recent program, students detailed their greatest anxieties in entering third year. The top five (highest = 1, and lowest = 10) were knowing enough medicine (2.23); performance and evaluation by supervisors (2.30); grading (3.51); taking care of patients (4.29); and time away from home, family, friends, and significant others (4.43).

––––––––

As students begin their fourth year of medical school, they experience increasing concerns about time. In addition to the broad-based education of the fourth year, students must attend to several other important matters: prepare for the residency search and match, which includes completing applications and amassing appropriate documentation; ready themselves for the USMLE Step 2; write personal statements and gather materials for the dean's letter; give their patients the proper attention; and find time for families and personal needs. Without the opportunity for reflection and assessment of priorities, they risk rushing headlong into the future and their residencies with only a vague idea of where they want to be on their career paths. To assist our fourth-year students, we issue booklets that cover various aspects of the residency programs and curricular offerings, hold numerous seminars, and schedule individual meetings with faculty advisors. Through these stratagems we seek in every way possible to build students' confidence, help them gain insight, and learn self-assessment. In addition, we hope to instill in students a realistic grasp of what they will encounter in the field of medicine. Many students have reported that they found these activities instrumental in helping them attain appropriate residencies.

At the graduation ceremony, to which we invite students' families and friends, we present prizes and awards for excellence in a variety of areas, including those that honor humanistic behavior. The dean discusses the tradition and meaning of the modified Hippocratic oath, and another speaker offers inspirational advice. We trust that this final act of honoring our graduates serves as a culminating experience in a continuum of professional development that will carry them forward as caring, compassionate physicians devoted to serving their patients.

––––––––

Not only do students contribute significantly to the events and ceremonies I have described above, they also assist in the admissions process. Using pre-established criteria that emphasize humanistic attributes, they help in recruiting, interviewing, and evaluating medical school applicants. In addition, we solicit our students' evaluations of our curriculum, and give serious consideration to their responses and suggestions for change. A variety of benefits accrue to the school as well as to the students: we gain their participation and assistance as well as the assurance that we are targeting their needs. Of tremendous importance is the fact that by valuing our students' contributions, we demonstrate our trust in their professional capabilities.

––––––––

Nearly every year students at Pritzker express interest in conducting a workshop or seminar on a topic they feel would enhance their understanding of an issue or help them function better as professionals. In almost every instance we have found the funds or means to comply. For instance, last year students reported that a faculty member's comments about a minority group had polarized their class. They determined to hold a diversity workshop to address this issue, and located an organization to host it. We set aside a day and requested all students to attend. Student feedback attested to the success of this activity. Attentiveness to students' needs and response with targeted events not only clarifies issues of concern, but forestalls potentially serious conflicts.

As another enhancement, we have a thanatologist available during gross anatomy classes to discuss with students their personal, emotional, and ethical concerns about death and dying. In order both to help students and to express respect, many schools have introduced memorial services for those persons whose bodies have been used as cadavers. Students participate in these services by sharing poems, singing, playing music, or in other ways expressing their gratitude for having received the gift of the cadaver as a tool for learning. Some institutions invite families of the deceased to the memorial services.

––––––––

All indicators point to the success of the aforementioned activities and events geared toward strengthening our students' professional growth. Candidates for admission to Pritzker often relate glowing reports from current students on the nurturing aspect of our school. Residents and faculty speak highly not only of our students' knowledge and skills, but also of their professionalism. Program directors consistently rank over 60 percent of each graduating class in the top

20 percent of all evaluated residents in terms of outstanding initiative, excellent attitudes about their work, excellent abilities to project the qualities of a "good" physician, excellent sensitivity to the psychosocial needs of patients, and high-quality relationships with other residents. Based on our success, I believe that all medical schools can successfully design many need-based activities for students that will greatly enhance their professional development.

The Informal Curriculum:
Mentoring, Social Activism, and Assessment

In examining the informal or hidden curriculum to discern where students encounter the most serious problems, medical school administrators and educators have focused on mistreatment by faculty and residents, particularly excessive workloads and inappropriate evaluations. Abuse and mistreatment have proven to be "a significant factor in making students more cynical about their educational experience and the practice of medicine" (Stern, 1996, p. 38). Students who suffer mistreatment lose their grasp of the humanistic principles we strive so hard to infuse and enhance. While educators endeavor to teach medical students the standards implicit in the modified Hippocratic oath, students do not always adopt these principles, in part because faculty and staff do not consistently demonstrate appropriate values.

Kassebaum and Cutler (1998) described several measures that could aid in the prevention of student maltreatment, including the following: establish standards for acceptable conduct in student-teacher relations; create educational programs for faculty to heighten their sensitivity to and awareness of the effects of student abuse; and create an office to investigate and manage reported incidents. Although we cannot control all aspects of this serious problem, we can at least better prepare our students in advance for the realities of the informal curriculum, and provide them with strategies for dealing with adversities. Fortunately, we have the support of the Liaison Committee on Medical Education (LCME), which has taken steps through its accreditation standards to support medical schools' attempts to create humane environments.

Turning to the positive side of the hidden curriculum, Hafferty points out that "the informal curriculum targets learning at the level of interpersonal interactions" (1998, p. 404). The most profound aspect of this interaction occurs in the impact that role models and mentors have on students. This finding makes it imperative that our doctors-in-training be treated with respect and compassion so they can preserve their own compassion and respect for their patients

(Stamos, 1996). Role models can also stimulate students' intellectual curiosity, instill a dedication to lifelong learning, and expand students' concept of professionalism. In addition, these individuals reflect strongly on the institution and ultimately on the practice of medicine.

Many advantages would accrue if each student could develop a relationship with a humanistic mentor. Because they interact with students on a more intimate level than role models, mentors can best nurture students' abilities. As Grady-Weliky, Kettyle, and Hundert note in another chapter of this book, faculty-member mentors must incorporate both personal and professional development in their relationship with students in order to effectively fulfill their half of the mentoring contract. The mentors who appear to do the best job are those who understand and empathize with the values and perspectives of today's students. Students who have been unsuccessful in resolving conflicts with faculty members pose a special challenge to medical educators. Because role models and mentors often lack the power to intercede, these students can easily become alienated from the educational process. We can best help students who find themselves in a conflicted situation by having administrative staff available who listen, treat them in a humanistic manner, *and* have sufficient stature to be heard on a student's behalf. Allowing for casual interchange between students without the presence of faculty has also proven quite valuable. Hundert's (1996) observations along these lines have led to Harvard's instituting student-to-student support systems that augment standard programs. These include peer counseling, resident assistants in the dormitories, anatomy lab discussion sessions, and various other discussion groups.

———

Many of today's students have an inherent orientation to social activism and a strong desire to advocate for the less fortunate in our society. Many cherish a sense of community and want to give back some of what they have gained. In fact, some feel so strongly about the importance of community work that they select medical schools that foster involvement in social causes. Both our institutions and our students benefit when students volunteer in community service activities in which they believe. Their experiences reinforce their leadership abilities and humanistic instincts, bolster their confidence, and furnish them with insight into their place in the field of medicine. Some of Pritzker's community outreach efforts include an HIV-prevention program, in which students visit schools to discuss the risk of HIV from unprotected sex and drug use, and a teen pregnancy prevention program which operates in the same manner.

In many instances over the years, Pritzker students have determined particular community needs and organized responsive programs. A prime example

Norma E. Wagoner

of this is the Community Health Initiative, in which students go to various community locations, including churches and subsidized housing units, to set up primary care clinics. Homeless women and children make up the majority of those who come for help in the form of basic health care and triage to other social and health care agencies. Another exceptionally successful venture has been the Adolescent Substance Abuse Prevention Program (ASAP), in which approximately 90 percent of our students elect to participate. The students designed this program, developed a curriculum module and workbook, and obtained funding from a local foundation to present it to fifth- and sixth-graders in Chicago. Medical students show the children actual human organs and demonstrate the effects of drug use. The Adolescent and Substance Abuse Prevention Program was one of eight chosen in the United States in 1999 to receive a national award from the Department of Health and Human Services for an outstanding grass-roots program. It was also chosen by the American Medical Student Association (AMSA) to serve as a national curriculum model for AMSA programs in United States medical schools. The Chicago public school system recently adopted the ASAP curriculum module for one of its educational offerings for fifth- and sixth-graders in the 1999–2000 academic year.

By enabling students to better understand themselves, gauge their own ethical beliefs and actions, and actively assess their own professional growth, we give them vital assistance in developing lifelong learning skills. Several former students have indicated how much they appreciated our advising them to keep a journal, and how helpful it was to look back and see their own progress. Journal writing proves especially beneficial during the third year, when students encounter new and intense stimuli, and the need for reflection becomes imperative. Encouraging students to reflect on their experiences and to analyze their emotional and ethical development ideally begets a lifelong habit of self-assessment.

Most evaluation instruments aim to measure achievement of educational objectives, and tend to be formulaic. In order to determine how well students are acquiring ethical principles, we need to assess more complex behaviors. We can accomplish this most effectively if we recruit peers, nurses, and other staff members to assist in the evaluation process. In fact, ABIM has already pioneered these practices at the residency level (1999). Although restricted staff time poses a limiting factor with large medical school classes, we must continue to explore ways of obtaining these important evaluations.

If we can succeed in doing this, the way would be paved for us to better modify student behavior by reinforcing their strengths, addressing infractions, and suggesting alternatives. Even the most compassionate students occasionally project unprofessional images. For instance, a shy student may appear uninterested, a candid student may appear as uncaring, a witty student as insensitive or even cruel. Encouraging students to self-evaluate and to share their findings with mentors would be beneficial. We can also design special workshops for students whose evaluations disclose problems with listening to or communicating with patients, staff members, and colleagues, or who aren't performing well as team members.

Hafferty argues that "one of the great challenges facing medical educators today lies in being willing and able to step back and assess just what messages are being created by and within the very structures they have developed and are responsible for" (1998, p. 404). By and large, medical schools do an excellent job of designing courses and clinical experiences that meet students' needs. However, we definitely need to assess and improve the informal curriculum. The LCME (1998) requires schools to offer programs to instill students with the ethical standards of a compassionate physician devoted to serving patients and the community. But it does not require that schools develop a continuum of activities and events to enhance students' professional development along the lines suggested in this chapter. One LCME requirement that would greatly promote professionalism is to expect schools to cite as an objective the inculcation of professionalism within the informal curriculum and, in conjunction with this, to state specific methods of evaluation.

Now that managed care has forced medical schools to extend their teaching and care of patients in the outpatient setting, care in community sites must now be much more fully appraised. Ten years ago our students acquired all their clinical experiences in the hospital. As they go out into the community and see the needs of their patients firsthand, their experiences not only open their eyes to the realities of their patients' lives, but position them better to become advocates for change. We can best capitalize on our students' experiences by listening to the recommendations they make based on their work. One very important outcome of community practice has been the students' realization that many patients seek some form of alternative care, including palliation and spiritual healing. An increasing number of patients want their physicians to pray with them. In response to these patient interests, medical schools have begun courses in alternative medicine, death and dying, and spirituality.

Another critical issue to be addressed involves the loss of physician autonomy, which has been described as a shift from "rugged individualism to entrepreneurial teamwork" (Souba, 1996, p. 4). Being an effective team member has become one of the most essential components of professionalism. Medical schools can do much more to instill the skills, attitudes, and ethical tenets that will enable students to communicate better and to establish solid working relationships with a diverse array of other professionals.

———

Students meet many obstacles on the long, difficult road to becoming a physician. Some succeed in maintaining their altruistic principles, avoiding selfish goals, and holding tightly to their calling. We can assist our students best by maintaining a keen awareness of what they learn as well as what we teach. Within the environment of the medical school, we must create a continuum of enhancing activities that both meet our students' needs and reinforce the professional values we honor.

FREDERICK A. MILLER
WILLIAM D. MELLON
with an afterword by HOWARD WAITZKIN

Experiencing Community Medicine during Residency

The La Mesa Housecleaning Cooperative

After several years of indoctrination in individually based, disease-oriented approaches, senior medical students may be unprepared to learn a population perspective. Residents, who encounter additional time demands and patient care responsibilities, present yet another challenge. The Community Health Partnerships program at the University of New Mexico (UNM), sponsored by the Kellogg Foundation and the New Mexico Department of Health, tried to foster the involvement of medical residents in community-oriented primary care (COPC) projects in local communities. A variety of activities developed from this collaboration, most of which have focused less on specific clinical outcomes than on a more global perspective of health. One of the major goals of the residents was to interact with a community and allow community members to define a project and its goals. Though unstated initially, residents' goals were to experience — as opposed to reading about — work in the community. They wanted to put theory into practice and learn by doing.

Involvement in the Kellogg Project thus facilitated three essential steps in teaching residents community medicine. Didactic sessions provided sufficient background to begin the work. Then the residents were able to go into the community and learn experientially. Finally, in evaluating the project, they were able to reflect on what was learned and to link theory with practice.

Prior to initiating the project, the residents discussed the expanded World Health Organization definition of health, which includes social, physical, economic, emotional, and spiritual well-being, in addition to the absence of disease. As this view has become more widely accepted in the medical community, there has been increasing recognition that the major causes of morbidity and mortality cannot be addressed simply in individual practitioners' offices. Among important recognized determinants or correlates of health are socioeconomic status and education (Hahn et al., 1995; Kaufman, Cooper, & McGee, 1997; Pappas, Queen, Hadden, & Fisher, 1993), social support and networks (Berkman, 1984; Eisenberg, 1979), self-efficacy and empowerment (Lawrance & McLeroy, 1986; Wallerstein, 1992), and community development and increased community capacity (Kretzman & McKnight, 1993). Along with an increased appreciation of these complex forces, practitioners interested in improving community health status have learned that health-promoting interventions imposed from the outside, without community ownership, are less likely to succeed or be sustained (Kretzman & McKnight, 1993).

With this understanding, two of us, both family practice residents at UNM, began a dialogue with a community about the problems they faced, with the intent of developing ideas for joint action. The notion of forming a cooperative grew out of these discussions. A review of the experience of successful cooperatives indicated that major health correlates such as socioeconomic status, education, empowerment, social support, and community development might be better addressed in such an activity, rather than through more traditional health promotion approaches.

A cooperative is any business organization that is owned and controlled by its members. The principles of cooperatives, as defined by the International Cooperative Alliance, include voluntary and open membership; democratic control by members; equitable and democratic control of capital; autonomy and independence; education, training, and information; cooperation among cooperatives; and concern for sustainable community development (Krimerman & Lindenfeld, 1992).

In their book *When Workers Decide* (1992), Krimerman and Lindenfeld highlight some of the advantages of cooperatives, both to workers and to the communities in which they reside. Weiss and Clamp's (1992) description of some of the advantages that relate to known health correlates includes the following:

Socioeconomic status/education. For workers, cooperatives offer a form of job protection, since the participants decide who is hired and fired. Profits are distributed equitably among all members, so if things go well workers tend to benefit from increased income. In the process of becoming managers as well as workers, cooperative members learn new skills, which not only add more reward to the work they do, but also provide them with lifelong assets to apply in other endeavors.

Social support and networks. Working together, members form support networks and learn the value and power of communal enterprises to accomplish more than can be accomplished individually.

Empowerment. In becoming owners and seeing a process through, members are more apt to develop confidence in themselves, and apply this confidence to other aspects of their lives.

Community development. Cooperatives are, by definition, locally owned and run. Therefore the money that is generated stays within the community, and the cooperative itself is often more responsive to community needs.

These benefits can lead to successful business ventures by creating motivated, educated, and activated worker-owners. In addition, the process of developing and sustaining a cooperative may have an impact upon the correlates of health previously mentioned.

————

The La Mesa Cooperative developed out of a collaboration between supporters from various disciplines and a group of approximately twelve Mexican immigrant women. The supporters included both of us (FAM and WDM), a community activist, a technical aid assistant who provided business advice and loans to women starting small businesses, and a teacher at La Mesa elementary school, where the children of the women in the cooperative were enrolled.

Following the passage of new immigration and welfare laws in 1996, the Kellogg Learner Group at UNM was concerned about possible adverse effects of the legislation on health and decided to focus on a community response. First they met with representatives of a community group trying to address Latino issues. The community activist and another coworker described in detail to the learner group the concerns they saw as most pressing within the immigrant community. The learner group also arranged community meetings with immigrant groups in Albuquerque to review key aspects of the new laws. One of these meetings was held at the La Mesa elementary school, where the participating teacher had organized a group of approximately one hundred Spanish-speaking parents with whom she had been working for over three years. We spoke with the group about their concerns regarding health in general, as well as how their access to care might be affected by the new laws. We asked the audience if there was any interest in forming a separate group to develop a community response to their situation and collated the names of those interested. A meeting was called for the following week, and the beginnings of a community dialogue took shape.

In the months prior to these meetings, the Kellogg group completed a partial needs assessment in that area of Albuquerque known as the Southeast Heights. They knew the area was composed mainly of immigrant groups, most having arrived only in the last five years. The majority were low-income families. Most services were available only for legal United States residents.

We started meeting with a group of low-income, Spanish-speaking, immigrant families, some of them undocumented. At this point our agenda was to find out from these families directly what concerned them most. Initially eight women showed up, and the first few meetings were spent discussing predominantly legal issues: What rights did people have if they were confronted by immigration officials? How should they respond to such a situation? What services were available to them, given their status? After several meetings, we posed a question to the group, adopting the perspective of community-oriented primary care (Kark, 1981): What are the major health problems facing your community, and what could you do about them? The women identified access to medical and dental care as a problem, including the inability to purchase medications and to pay for lab tests and treatments. They also mentioned their fears of going to the county-supported university hospital because they had been unable to pay prior debts for services received there.

However, the women unanimously concluded that the greatest barrier to healthier lives for their families and community was economic in origin: they needed jobs. If they had money, they could pay for visits to the doctor, medicines, and treatments. They could also pay for housing, clothing, food, and school supplies — all of which they saw as major factors affecting their health and well-being.

The supporters (the community activist, technical aid assistant, teacher, and both of us) suggested a cooperative, and the women responded very favorably to the idea. It seemed like an obvious solution. But then, what type of cooperative? The idea of a housecleaning cooperative surfaced. It required little initial investment for supplies, drew on skills the women felt they already had, and in the experience of women who had worked in private cleaning companies, could be very lucrative.

From that point on, meetings became more focused. The technical aid assistant presented the basic tasks required to start a business. A woman from a successful sewing cooperative in Albuquerque came to discuss the history of her group. The group arranged a site visit to see this cooperative in action. The women began inviting guests of their own, including a woman with her own cleaning business and another who spoke about selling cleaning products, to discuss details of their work.

As the project progressed, the group arranged various activities outside the meetings. A local priest was very helpful in obtaining school supplies for the women's children. He also set up several meetings for spiritual reflection at the church. Some women went to more formal English classes. The teacher-supporter facilitated paperwork for driver's licenses for some of the women, and the women who did not know how to drive began taking driving lessons.

At the time of this writing, the cooperative is in operation at a modest pace. Each woman is currently working one to three jobs a week. With our help, along with some medical students doing a one-month community project, the women received a thousand-dollar grant from the Kellogg project community board for a phone line and office operations. The women subsequently received another grant of five thousand dollars from the local chapter of Catholic Human Development to buy a used van and help pay for the driving lessons.

Perhaps the most surprising outcome was the change in the women's lives. Virtually all the women obtained jobs directly or indirectly through the cooperative. One woman who already had legal residency papers originally joined the cooperative to help take care of children. Through the meetings she discovered an administrative talent. She took a job cleaning rooms in a motel and within several months became the motel's manager of cleaning services. Two other women in the cooperative began to work for her, cleaning rooms. Another woman began her own business selling roasted corn door to door. Two others received payments from the state for home daycare.

All the women were open about the changes in their lives since joining the cooperative. One issue comprised their evolving relationships with their husbands, many of whom were not employed full time. As the women worked more hours, the husbands took on more domestic responsibilities. The men's traditional authority in the households shifted. At one meeting, the woman who managed cleaning services in a motel spontaneously said, "When I first began this cooperative, my husband told me if I got GED [high school equivalency certification], he would leave me. Now, as the commercial says, 'the rules have changed.' Now, he works for me."

The schoolteacher participating in the group also thrived in her role. Nominated by the supporters for her community work, she was selected to receive a prestigious award as an outstanding female leader and role model in the Hispanic community. Like doctors who work beyond the exam room, Edna became more involved in extracurricular activities as she saw the importance of addressing her students' needs beyond the classroom. From her work in the cooperative, Edna felt that she was focusing more on the sources of productive change. She has said that projects in community development, such as the cooperative, moved in the direction she wanted to pursue with the parents of her students.

The cooperative's path was not completely smooth. At times attendance at the meetings dropped off. At one point a very heated conflict erupted, splitting the cooperative into two factions. The issue ultimately centered on trust; the woman operating the phones, who was not a member but was paid by the cooperative for her bilingual capacities, was accused of not distributing jobs equitably. A local nun offered her services as a facilitator, and at an emotional meeting the women agreed to move forward together. We sometimes feared that the cooperative might not continue without external support. However, the tears these women shed as the conflict unfolded and began to resolve left no doubt of their emotional investment in the cooperative, and their desire to see it succeed. All the woman declared on several occasions that they will leave whatever job they are doing as soon as the cooperative can provide work full time.

We found our involvement in this project to be a very rich experience. While thus far the cooperative has not earned large sums of money, it has far exceeded our expectations. If the cooperative had stalled and fallen apart, we would still have learned many important lessons. What follows is a discussion of how the time invested in the project proved valuable to both us and the cooperative members. We then discuss how our experience fits within the curriculum of the family practice residency program. In conclusion, we speculate on how the lessons learned from this experience might be generalized to other settings for health professionals in training.

To obtain feedback after nine months in the project, we conducted a modest process evaluation. We held structured interviews with each woman in the cooperative and with each of the supporters (the community activist, the teacher, and the technical aid assistant), and we conducted a focus-group discussion with several women. Our intention was to elicit perceptions about the project's progress, to clarify goals, and to learn in what way we as medical providers were contributing to the process. The information we obtained was helpful in discovering subtle ways in which our presence affected the cooperative. In addition, the process of doing the evaluation itself became a stimulus for both the women and the supporters to reflect on the project and to renew their commitment with clearer objectives.

Through discussion with the women and the supporters, it became clear that our being health professionals, that is, physicians, was no more important than other aspects of our interactions with the group. Many of the women mentioned that we became a source of encouragement to them by asking questions about their lives, by listening, and by showing concern.

To the other supporters, the presence of two physicians at the meetings provided an important source of hope for the cooperative. The fact that we too saw this process as important helped the women to believe in it. One of the other supporters also pointed out that forming the cooperative helped decrease the gap between providers in the hospital and the people they served in the community. Everyone agreed that the participation of health care providers was significant because they were respected members of the community, like teachers, community activists, priests, or economic advisors. As health care providers we were viewed as trustworthy individuals with sincere intentions.

It was crucial that the supporters not assume too much authority if the women eventually were to take control of the cooperative. However, there were points in the process, particularly during the early phases, when substantial direction was needed. The supporters, including us, helped provide this direction, particularly in the organization of meetings. Early on, the unfocused jumping among topics seemed inefficient, but we generally stayed quiet and observed, not wanting to impose our administrative style or culturally and professionally biased views on how to conduct a meeting. However, when we asked the cooperative members at various times if they wanted us to contribute some regimentation to the flow of the meetings, the feedback was quite positive. Thereafter, when structure was noticeably lacking, one of us might ask for everyone's attention, facilitate the construction of an agenda, write it on a poster board, and then gently remind people to stick to the topic at hand when the discussion began to stray.

Some issues unique to health care providers arose. One involved providing medical advice. In the early meetings, the women mentioned medical problems, many centering around access to care. We responded by asking to speak with those questioners after the meeting, thus keeping our role as physicians quite informal. In addition, as professionals we held knowledge and experience concerning economic and professional institutions and infrastructure (e.g., finding grant money, recruiting a lawyer), advantages that became crucial when external assistance was needed.

In sum, becoming an effective supporter has meant unlearning many orientations that we had been taught as health care providers, particularly as physicians. Instead of demonstrating our knowledge, we tried to become more adept at listening and learning along with others. Instead of dominating the process, we found benefit in restricting our participation. Thus, instead of encountering powerful authority figures, cooperative members appreciated a sincere expression of concern at the human level. Above all, we learned that effectiveness in this process required flexibility. The process of organizing did not build linearly, step by step. Instead, we learned patience to allow the process to evolve gradually, even though at times more assertiveness was needed. Eventually we developed a sense of what the group needed at a given time, and the ability to assess realistically what they themselves could provide.

Frederick A. Miller and William D. Mellon with Howard Waitzkin

We initially were attracted to this project because it allowed for direct contact with community members. Both of us had been exposed to theory about community-based work and had worked in communities before medical school. However, we were unsure how our participation would unfold in our new role as physicians. Working over time with the cooperative, we began to have a sense of community members' lives, their priorities and exigencies, and their perception of us as physicians. Thus our learning was highly experiential.

From the beginning, we had few expectations for this project; our objective was to work with community members. The pace and evolution of a community activity can be quite different from the relentless deadlines of an academic center. For medical professionals, accustomed to tangible results and linear progress, it seemed at times that this work was a poor investment of our "valuable" time. To keep doing the work, we learned to value independent learning.

Perhaps the greatest insight we gained into these women's lives concerned the insulation from disorder and misfortune that wealth and privilege provide. Organizing meetings was a constant struggle. The women's ability to arrive depended on a host of factors beyond their control. Most of them came from households with many people and one car, and the women usually were not the drivers. Being able to arrive at a meeting meant that no child got sick, no one was late coming home from work, no one else needed to be picked up, and the car, usually secondhand and well used, did not break down.

Beyond that were the basic uncertainties of everyday life. Several times women could not attend meetings because they urgently needed to do a job to get enough money to pay that month's rent. One woman's son was deported. The children of several other women were involved in violent incidents. One woman and her entire family were evicted. Two others would have been, if the teacher participant had not helped them with the rent. We learned that the people of this community lived far more on a day-to-day basis than we had ever imagined was possible. Investing gradually for the future, we learned, becomes very difficult when one is trying to survive until next week.

Once everyone managed to get there, running the meeting presented a challenge. The women were responsible for about twenty children. For a period of time, the cooperative met in a gymnasium so the women could keep an eye on the children while they played. However, with so much noise, balls bouncing on the meeting notes or on people's heads, the group opted to move to the Kellogg program office, which had a place where the children could play in a room separated from us by windows.

Another challenge involved negotiating the cultural and gender differences between ourselves — white, male professionals — and the cooperative members — low-income, Hispanic mothers. We became aware of how medical training had constructed the lens through which we saw the women. In this process, we struggled with tendencies to perceive the women as less rational and less efficient than we were, as well as characterized by unhealthy behaviors that needed to be changed for their own benefit. Being present in the neighborhood and not in the hospital, we had to adjust our attitudes and behavior. As we came to understand the demands in the women's lives, their responsibilities, the love they showed toward their children, and the dignity they maintained despite enormous stresses, we were reminded of important values we had momentarily forgotten.

During the meetings, even without clear goals, our agenda tended to be businesslike, while the women would interject talk about "nonbusiness" matters during discussions. We noticed in the beginning that the women were unaccustomed to having meetings with a planned agenda, with abstract topics to guide discussions chronologically, and rigid time limits. Topics seemed to flow in and out of discussion somewhat randomly, the meetings started late and ended late, and to us, not much appeared to be accomplished. After observing for some time, we realized that the women were becoming as frustrated as we were and welcomed the structure we and the other supporters could provide. In this way, the cultural and gender gaps were bridged by efforts on both sides showing mutual respect.

A difficult lesson was seeing how frustrating the women's situations could be. Conflicts tended to break out during the lulls in progress for the cooperative. People were not earning the money that they needed desperately to pay essential bills. In frustration, they sometimes lashed out at those in the cooperative who were doing somewhat better. On the other hand, those women who were beginning to do better economically themselves appeared at times to put distance between themselves and those struggling on rungs just a bit lower on the economic ladder.

We found these insights important, as workers in the community and also as health care providers. It was not hard to imagine how the same barriers that made it difficult for the women to get to a meeting and to run it efficiently also made it difficult for them to be "good" patients who take their medicines, do their exercises, and keep their appointments. In helping them after the meetings with their personal health concerns, we learned still more about these problems. It was difficult for the women to have access to services at the hospital because of lack of money, language barriers, and mistrust of large institutions. We felt that our role as intermediaries between the women and the health care system was at least as helpful to them as anything else we contributed to the cooperative.

––––––––––

The educational philosophy at UNM in the Department of Family and Community Medicine has led to opportunities and flexibility for residents to pursue interests on an individualized basis. The department has a reputation for focusing on population-based health issues and has facilitated a network of training sites for medical students and residents outside the hospital and throughout the state. The community medicine curriculum in the residency program reflects these values. Residents are encouraged to think about health problems from a public health perspective. Curriculum flexibility allows residents to utilize time and resources at the university and the New Mexico Department of Health for their projects.

The family practice curriculum requires a community project during the second and third years of residency. Residents can choose to spend a month working intensively on the project, or can spread it out over two years, working one half-day each week on the average. Since the last two years of family practice residency include mostly outpatient rotations, arranging a half-day away from clinic is feasible. During inpatient rotations, continuity becomes more difficult, and meetings must be scheduled at night, or with more frequency in subsequent months. During some rotations at rural sites, it is occasionally possible to attend community events, but usually the work simply has to wait until one returns.

The community medicine curriculum has a coordinator, who identifies possible projects and links residents with activities along their lines of interest. Each resident is required to choose a project and to write a proposal, to which the curriculum coordinator responds with suggestions. At the end of residency, all residents submit reports. A faculty member serves as advisor for each resident.

There are two tracks in the community medicine curriculum: basic and advanced. The goals for the basic curriculum are to learn the fundamentals of several areas: epidemiology and public health; clinical prevention services; partnerships with existing public health services; doctor-patient communication and social, cultural, and behavioral issues in the context of disease; and working with local communities. The advanced curriculum is for those residents interesting in pursuing their interest in community medicine further. In conjunction with classwork in the M.P.H. program, these residents work with public health officials throughout New Mexico. Upon graduation they receive a certificate of public health, which acknowledges the additional training they have had and which can be applied for credit toward an M.P.H. degree.

Residents' projects have varied. Several residents have implemented a violence prevention curriculum in a local high school. Others have done health education in the primary schools. One was involved in a health needs assessment for immigrant, uninsured Hispanics. Two others helped set up a statewide domestic violence prevention program. While some residents spend extensive time in their community projects, others are less interested in doing so and put together a project late in residency, or do clinical work in a school or homeless shelter for the community medicine project. In addition to the community medicine curriculum coordinator, numerous faculty members in the department have ongoing community projects themselves and are open to working with residents when approached.

The Kellogg program has served as a focal point for bringing together nurses, social workers, law students, and faculty members interested in doing interdisciplinary work promoting healthier communities. This backdrop was helpful for the La Mesa project. We felt encouraged to do a community project and to take time away from clinical medicine for the needed activities. The program was also quite open to a project that was not within the traditional purview of public health.

In terms of didactic learning, we both had done classwork during medical school in medical anthropology, looking at cross-cultural issues in health care. Throughout the course of residency, during grand rounds and special lectures, the family practice program provided several sessions on community-oriented primary care as well as the social determinants of health. Finally, the Kellogg project itself tried to bring in speakers tailored to learners' interests as different projects unfolded. Thus, we attended sessions on how to do community organizing, how to conduct needs assessments, and how to do surveys. We also received legal briefings on immigration and welfare law, as well as on the passage of bills through the state legislature. Presenters included a local community organizer, faculty members in the Department of Family and Community Medicine and the M.P.H. program, as well as an immigration lawyer and officials from the state Department of Health.

While we did not look to any single faculty member to direct our work, we were able to draw on abundant faculty support when the time came to write up the project. Faculty members were very supportive with feedback and suggestions which helped to maintain a clear focus in the work. Moreover, the act of doing a process evaluation and writing up the progress of the cooperative, as mentioned above, helped us reflect on what we were doing and resulted in everyone — ourselves and the women in the cooperative — taking the work they were doing more seriously.

Most residents in the program took on more traditional public health activities. Few residents have expressed interest in taking over this project. Potential successors are probably constrained by the requirement of speaking Spanish, the less-direct health focus, and a preference for starting their own projects. However, the cooperative itself has sufficient support and momentum to continue without resident involvement.

———

We are entering a new era in popular conceptions of health. The expanded framework of individual and community health, as exemplified by the World Health Organization's definition, reflects a growing understanding of the many factors which support well-being and contribute to illness. Health professionals and the systems in which they function are being forced to rethink traditional approaches to community health promotion and to recognize the necessity of developing new strategies in the education of health professionals.

Our experience with this project emphasized various skills, essential in doing effective work in community medicine, but many of which are given little attention in medical school or residency training. Traditionally, the disease-oriented approach to medicine has dominated medical education and continues to do so. In an article about involving primary care physicians in community empowerment, Eng, Salmon, and Mullan (1992) argue that most physicians are not trained in the skills necessary for effective community empowerment, and that many skills of physicians run contrary to the principles of facilitating communities to take control of their circumstances. COPC aims to expand the analysis of health and society, to highlight the social sciences in medicine in order to gain a better understanding of the factors which have impact upon individuals and communities, and ultimately to cultivate the will of society to address these factors.

The project also taught us some lessons about doing community-oriented primary care. Kark (1981) suggests that COPC proceeds in stages: (1) data collection and the development of a community health diagnosis, (2) planning an intervention, (3) implementation, and (4) surveillance, evaluation, and planning for future action. However, the experience of community-oriented primary care does not always follow such a clear-cut, linear pathway. In the case of La Mesa, the needs assessment remained far from comprehensive but rather elicited community members' concerns through direct dialogue. The evaluation, meanwhile, occurred during the implementation stage. Instead of focusing on a particular health issue, we looked at the women's overall life concerns and developed a project with the women's main priorities in mind.

Given the time constraints of graduate medical education, where can one find the time to learn the skills necessary for effective community work? The answer lies, perhaps, in the pace of learning. We had one half-day a week for work on community projects longitudinally. Although this was not a large amount of time, over two years it provided the basis for an ongoing dialectic of action and reflection that led to fruitful learning. Another helpful tactic was to team up with one or more other residents so that when one is doing a rotation away or is on call, the other can try to adjust his or her schedule so that at least one learner can attend important community or project events.

We conclude, based on these experiences, that the key ingredients needed for potentially successful projects include the following:

Protected time — one half-day per week over two years

Faculty willing to support the work

Formal education — didactic sessions and readings in cross-cultural issues and community organizing

Learners who believe this work is worthwhile — convinced either by example, by readings that discuss the major social determinants of health, or by brief immersion experiences (learners must see why this work is a valuable use of their time; otherwise the incessant demands of learning clinical medicine will always pull them away)

A focus more on process than concrete outcomes

Work implemented through community leaders who can link learners to community residents

Work organized in pairs or teams, to achieve a consistent presence despite difficult schedules

Opportunity for reflection — via a final report and/or group discussion, to think about what was learned and to discuss the congruencies and disparities of theory and practice

The act of going into a community, preferably accompanied by a liaison who is trusted and known in the community, with an open mind and without preconceptions or the belief one already has all the answers, can begin the process of community dialogue. If a health care provider in training is prepared with sufficient background to appreciate the importance of doing this work, much can be learned from engaging in this process as an equal party with other community members. McKnight (1997) summarizes this approach well: "To enhance community health, we need a new breed of modest health professionals, people who respect the integrity and wisdom of citizens and their associations" (p. 24).

Afterword

This report summarizes two family practice residents' efforts to help a community-based group of poor and undocumented women in their attempt to start a housecleaning cooperative. Why would this project interest medical educators?

For faculty members committed to teaching the principles of primary care, community medicine, and the social sciences, the challenges of medical education often are daunting. While innovative programs can sometimes excite trainees to expand their interests and change their career direction, teachers who work in this area know that such successes remain difficult to predict. A meaningful goal in this arena, as in other arenas of clinical medicine, is "to do no harm." That is, it is important to provide a supportive educational context so that trainees who enter our programs already committed to primary care and community-oriented work do not give up this commitment during the stresses of clinical education. From this viewpoint, much of our responsibility as educators rests in assuring that trainees do not lose their initial idealism — a sad process that affects many medical students and residents who become dissuaded from their initial commitments because of unsupportive training experiences.

The authors of this chapter are gifted physicians who entered the study of medicine largely to pursue their earlier commitments in the realm of community-based activism and social justice. Rick Miller and Bill Mellon had participated actively in organizing efforts and clinical work within low-income and minority communities before they entered their residencies. As residents, they took the initiative to continue this community-oriented work, which they continue to pursue now that they have completed their residency training. Rick, Bill, and people like them bring with them the experience, knowledge, and commitment that increase the likelihood that their eventual careers in medicine will manifest the values that led them into medicine initially — unless these values become thwarted by their experiences during training. Aside from the goal of positively influencing learners who enter their training not fully committed, we as educators bear responsibility for assuring that learners who are fully committed, like Rick and Bill, do not become disillusioned or burned out.

Faculty members at the University of New Mexico (UNM) have struggled for many years to develop and implement programs that encourage medical students and residents to practice primary care, especially in rural areas. The UNM School of Medicine has achieved a series of curricular innovations that have encompassed problem-based learning, learner-oriented small-group tutorials, decentralized learning experiences at primary care sites in underserved areas, and protected time to pursue community-based projects (see, for example, Kaufman et al., 1996). These efforts have attracted some acclaim, both nationally and internationally. Partly because of its reputation for educational innovation and a supportive environment for primary care and community medicine, UNM has attracted many medical students and residents who already have clear commitments and accomplishments in these arenas. As a relative newcomer to UNM (director of community medicine starting in 1997), I can take no credit for the school's achievements, but I certainly have benefited from the opportunities that the educational environment provides for learners, who clearly encompass the faculty as well as students and residents.

The Kellogg-supported program to which Rick and Bill refer has provided a base for interdisciplinary learning among residents, medical students, nursing students, and trainees in other allied health professions. As Rick and Bill point out, the Kellogg program encouraged them to meet with other learners and with faculty advisors in carrying out a community-based project. Faculty responsible for the Kellogg program have tried to maximize freedom for committed learners to pursue projects of their choosing. For that reason, the project that Rick and Bill describe — which aimed to enhance a community group's attempts toward economic development rather than narrow medical or public health goals — received enthusiastic support from faculty advisors and peers. Other educational contexts may have proven less supportive for this innovative project, which superficially seemed to bear little relationship to the traditional goals of medicine and public health.

Aside from the freedom and time to pursue an unusual community project, the UNM environment provided an opportunity for the learners to experience firsthand a situation with profound implications for health outcomes. By encouraging the women's cooperative to pursue economic development rather than more restricted medical or public health goals, the residents witnessed a process by which community members intuitively reached a conclusion that finally is gaining academic acknowledgment: that economic conditions are more important as a determinant of health outcomes than are medical or public health interventions (see Hahn et al., 1995; Krieger & Sidney, 1996; Montgomery, Kiela, & Pappas, 1996; Pappas et al., 1997; Pappas, Queen, Hadden, & Fisher, 1993). Working with undocumented, very low income women, the residents facilitated the women's efforts to improve their economic conditions as a primary goal.

Economic development, for the women in the housecleaning cooperative, became a precondition for other improvements in their quality of life, mental health, and physical health. The potential benefits of economic development for health outcomes remained implicit throughout the time that the residents worked with the community. Yet, by focusing on the improvement of economic conditions as the goal of a community medicine project, the residents aimed to foster changes that had a higher probability of contributing to positive health outcomes than many or most narrowly defined health interventions. This profound characteristic of the project reinforced the residents' earlier learning experiences, deepening rather than thwarting their fundamental commitments during the vicissitudes of their clinical training. In this sense, their mentors' attempts to foster this unusual community-based learning seemed to accomplish something more than doing no harm.

ACKNOWLEDGMENTS

Support for the La Mesa project came in part from the Kellogg Foundation Grant for Community Health Partnerships awarded to the UNM Health Sciences Center for forming interdisciplinary efforts in the postgraduate programs of medicine and nursing to form sustainable community projects. Edna Alvarado provided important comments which have been incorporated into this paper.

DONALD WASYLENKI

NIALL BYRNE

BARBARA McROBB

Community-Oriented Medical Education

The Toronto Experience

A principal concern of medical educators during the past decade has been whether modern physicians are being trained to respond to society's changing health needs. Some medical educators describe medical education as "a public trust" and argue that in several critical areas academic medicine is not fulfilling its fundamental social responsibility to improve the health of the public (Schroeder, Jones, & Showstack, 1989), including the obligation to provide society with appropriately prepared physicians responsive to its health care needs. Richards also describes "a gap between what medical education prepares physicians to do and what society needs" (1990, p. 97). He describes a "social contract" between medical education and society, the fulfilment of which, in return for public support, involves the discovery and transmission of knowledge which will address society's problems. A need exists, he concludes, for medical education to renew its social contract, and he recommends that this be effected through the linking of medical education with its external environment — the community itself. Murray also contends that too often the medical profession's attempts to serve society are narrow and poorly informed (in LeBourdais, 1994). He points out that the public has become more sophisticated and increasingly aware of the importance of broad health determinants such as lifestyle, diet, stress, and family dysfunction, whereas medical schools provide little or no exposure to these issues.

At an international conference held in 1990, The Medical School's Mission and the Population's Health, medical educators from Canada, the United Kingdom, the United States, and Australia convened to focus upon the question of the medical school's responsibility for understanding and meeting the health care needs of the community (White & Connelly, 1992). In a paper titled "The Social Contract and the Medical School's Responsibilities," Inui (1992) argues for the teaching of medicine in locales other than inpatient wards and a greater emphasis on the clinical relevance of population-based information and perspectives. These themes are developed in several major reports on undergraduate medical education.

In the United States the GPEP Report, *Physicians for the Twenty-First Century* (Association of American Medical Colleges, 1984), recommends that "medical students' general professional education should include an emphasis on the physician's responsibility to work with individual patients and communities to promote health and prevent disease" (p. 3). *Medical Education in Transition*, the report of the Robert Wood Johnson Foundation Commission on Medical Education, includes a recommendation that medical schools expand the context of training beyond tertiary care hospitals to a variety of settings in the community (Marston & Jones, 1992). The report of the Pew Health Professions Commission, *Healthy America: Practitioners for 2005* (1991), includes among competencies for the year 2005 care for the community's health (Shugars, O'Neil, & Bade, 1991). This entails "a broad understanding of the determinants of health such as environment, socioeconomic conditions, behaviors, medical care and genetics and the ability to work with others in the community to integrate a range of services and activities that promote, protect and improve health" (p. 18).

Similar themes emerge from documents from the United Kingdom. In particular, a report issued by the King's Fund Centre, *Community-Based Teaching*, presents a detailed rationale for the development of community-based medical education and provides a series of examples of community-oriented learning experiences in U.K. medical schools (Towle, 1992). A survey of medical undergraduate community-based teaching in U.K. universities by McCrorie, Lefford, and Perrin (1993) netted eighty-three courses from the twenty-eight medical schools surveyed. In Canada, the report "Toward Integrated Medical Resource Policies for Canada" recommends that undergraduate curricula shift the location of training away from urban tertiary care hospitals and that affiliation agreements for medical education be developed with a broader range of institutions, community locations, and clinical faculty (Barer & Stoddart, 1992). In Ontario, the Educating Future Physicians for Ontario (EFPO) project (1993) has the goal of making medical education in Ontario more responsive to the changing needs of society: increasing the time medical students spend in the community will provide them with a better understanding of the needs of the community and a greater awareness of available community resources. The report also points out that "people in the community expect physicians to help their community be healthier" and recommends that undergraduate medical curricula include concepts and information regarding all determinants of health.

Internationally, the 1993 World Summit on Medical Education included among its recommendations participation of communities in medical education (Walton, 1993). The recommendation states that "community participation will encourage interdisciplinary learning and multiprofessional teamwork. A larger community role in the educational process will increase the accountability and relevance of medical education, enhance community compliance with health initiatives and promote development and improved health." In addition, the report recommended an expansion of "real-world settings" for medical education and an increased commitment of universities to population-based medical education. Finally, the international Network of Community-Oriented Education Institutions for the Health Sciences has been in existence since 1979 (Schmidt, Neufeld, Nooman, & Ogunbode, 1991). The network consists of 56 full-member institutions, 115 associate members, and 61 corresponding members, scattered around the globe — in Africa, North America, the eastern Mediterranean, Europe, Southeast Asia, and the western Pacific. The network has five primary goals:

Helping membership institutions realize the importance of community-
    oriented learning and appropriate instructional methods
Strengthening of faculty capacities related to community-based education
Developing technologies, approaches, methodologies, and tools appropriate
    to a community-oriented curriculum, such as problem-based learning
Promoting population concepts in the health services system and the
    curriculum
Assisting institutions in countries having a political intent to introduce
    innovation in the training of health personnel, with the ultimate goal of
    improving health care and contributing to the achievement of "Health
    for All"

In addition to international network events held throughout the world at regular internals, a regular network newsletter contains information from member institutions.

With these objectives and recommendations in mind when the Faculty of Medicine at the University of Toronto embarked upon undergraduate curriculum reform in 1990, they decided to incorporate a "community half-day" experience throughout the first and second medical school years. For one half-day each week during the first two years of medical school, all 252 students in each class would spend time learning in the community as an important dimension of a broadened approach to medical education, embracing the evolving determinants-of-health paradigm.

Donald Wasylenki, Niall Byrne, and Barbara McRobb

Course Initiation

Course development was beset by problems early in the process. Although a planning committee was formed, and it produced a series of community learning objectives, faculty had difficulty in imagining how such a large group of students could be provided with learning experiences in the community, even though Toronto has a population of approximately 2.5 million, with hundreds of community-based health and social service agencies. The difficulty seemed to lie in moving from the traditional approach of having students spend time in doctors' offices to a new approach more in keeping with community and population health perspectives. A second problem involved lack of leadership. As the implementation date for the new curriculum approached, it became clear that there was no individual prepared to assume the position of course director for the community half-day and to take responsibility for planning and implementation. Up until approximately three months before the curriculum was to be implemented, the group attempting to plan the community half-day was chaired by the coordinator of curriculum development, acting on an interim basis. This difficulty in recruiting a course director was partially related to a third difficulty. The faculty had not been prepared to allocate sufficient resources to support an undertaking of this magnitude, involving coordination of several hundred community placements each semester. Potential candidates for the course directorship were appropriately skeptical of the faculty's commitment to the community half-day concept, given the reluctance to provide adequate support.

In an atmosphere of relative crisis, roughly four months before the new curriculum was to begin, a full-time administrator was employed for the community half-day experience who in turn recruited a course director. This was an individual whose academic background was in community psychiatry and who therefore had experience in working with community agencies, primarily in the mental health field.

Following the commitment of resources and the recruitment of a course director, a formal course-planning committee was established. This committee was multidisciplinary with representation from the faculty, the community, and eventually the medical student class. Committee members met weekly for several hours throughout the summer to organize an initial community half-day experience for the fall term, as part of the launching of the new curriculum in September 1992. The committee quickly decided that the emphasis should be on providing students with stimulating community learning experiences and that the new course would be entitled Health, Illness, and the Community (HIC).

Faced with the challenge of quickly organizing community learning experiences for 252 students, the course-planning committee forged an educational alliance with the Home Care Program for Metropolitan Toronto (HCPMT). The HCPMT is the largest component of Ontario's provincial Home Care Program. HCPMT coordinates the provision of in-home health and social services throughout Metropolitan Toronto for individuals who require more than standard ambulatory care but less than hospitalization. It is one of the largest home health-care programs in the world and, on any given day, roughly twenty thousand patients are registered. This extensive and very modern health care agency had never before been utilized to educate medical students. Senior management staff at HCPMT were eager to participate in helping to develop the HIC course; they were aware of the rapid shift from hospital to community care and of the need for physicians to become more knowledgeable about their own and other community agencies. HCPMT was also ideally equipped to absorb a large number of medical students into a sophisticated coordination network.

Thus the original HIC course, which began in October 1992, involved first-year medical students, in pairs, accompanying home-care service providers throughout Metropolitan Toronto and observing, in the first weeks of medical school, a broad array of individuals coping with illness and disability at home, rather than in a tertiary care hospital. Faculty recruits led tutorial groups of six students to discuss the experiences they were having in the home care program. For many students, these experiences were eye-opening. Following two half-days of accompanying home care providers and a debriefing tutorial, each pair of students spent two half-days visiting one patient in the home care program at home, to gain an in-depth understanding of the experience of illness and disability in the community. This experience involved the recruitment of 126 patients through the home care program. A second debriefing tutorial followed, and then each pair of students prepared an oral presentation on some aspect of the community experience, which they presented to their tutors and tutorial group. Finally, each individual student submitted an essay on an issue related to health care in the community. Topics included the maintenance of autonomy, team functioning in the community, and the issue of competence; most essays utilized observed clinical material to illustrate important conceptual issues. Students received a numerical mark based upon attendance and participation and the quality of presentations and essays. Although the students performed extremely well in the course, there was dissatisfaction expressed during the initiation period with the requirement that students travel about the city and interact with nonmedical health care providers. Students had difficulty in understanding how this type of learning related to becoming a doctor.

Donald Wasylenki, Niall Byrne, and Barbara McRobb

Course Components

Five years later the HIC course in its fully developed state consists of three distinct components. Component one, Health Care in the Community, is part of the first semester of the first year. Component two, Promoting Health in the Community, occurs in the second semester of the first year. Component three, Achieving Health in the Community, occupies all of the second medical year. Each component takes place one half-day per week.

The first component, Health Care in the Community, begins in September and ends in mid January. It has been built upon the original home-care experience and involves strong educational partnerships among the faculty, the Home Care Program for Metropolitan Toronto, and sixteen inner-city schools. The overall goal of this component is to expose students to experiences of illness and disability in the community, to the functioning of community-based multidisciplinary teams, and to health issues faced by children in inner-city schools.

This first component begins with a large-group symposium on Canada's health care system to help students understand the importance of developing a community perspective. Prominent physicians introduce the course, and students learn about the evolution of the health care system and the current shift to community care; the importance of understanding health determinants such as gender, culture, and economic resources; and, finally, how the system must change in order to survive. Then the students break into groups of six, meet their tutors, and receive and begin to discuss their field-work assignments. Each tutorial group has both a medical and a nonmedical tutor to emphasize HIC's interdisciplinary orientation and to provide differing perspectives. For the next four weeks the students participate in one of two streams. Half of the students begin with the home-care field experience, going out in pairs for two consecutive weeks with a home-care service provider and/or coordinator. During this time they may encounter between six and twelve clinical situations in peoples' homes. Following this, each pair of students visits an individual home-care patient to understand further the experience of illness in the community. The other half of the class enters the inner-city schools stream, which begins with a symposium on children as a population. This is followed by an orientation session to prepare students to address health issues in the school environment. Then each pair of students spends three half-days in an inner-city elementary-school classroom, carrying out exercises to explore health-related issues. The final half-day is a health teaching session presentation by the medical students to the children in the school classroom.

Following this first block of field experiences, students attend a second large-group symposium on the role of the physician, presented by physicians who exemplify changing patterns of practice. Topics include international health; the physician as social activist; women's issues; and the importance of culture as a health determinant. The following week, which is week eight of the first semester, students reconvene in their small-group tutorials to discuss their field experiences. The second half of the tutorial focuses on multidisciplinary teamwork and the role of the physician as a team member. The students then return to the field for another four weeks and switch streams, so that those who completed the home care experience go to inner-city schools and vice versa. Week fourteen is a second small-group tutorial, where students once again discuss their experiences and work on a series of exercises related to social justice and resource allocation for health care. After a week to prepare presentations in pairs on an important health issue arising out of their field experience, each student submits an essay on a topic related to health care in the community. The first-semester numerical mark continues to be a composite of attendance, participation, and quality of presentations and essays.

––––––––––

In the second semester of the first year, which begins in February and ends in May, the focus shifts from the provision of health care in the community to health promotion. The overall goal of the second semester course, Promoting Health in the Community, is to help students understand broad health determinants and to begin to identify and develop health promotion strategies in the community. The organization of the second semester involves educational partnerships with approximately 150 community agencies from each of four broad networks, including drug and alcohol programs, community health centers, child and family services, and elderly persons' centers.

The second semester begins with a symposium on the determinants of health. A representative from each of the four networks discusses the importance of health determinants, after which students receive reading materials and their field assignments. Each pair of students begins field work by spending four half-days in one agency in one of the networks learning about health determinants. For example, a pair of students may learn how programs for the elderly help to maintain both morale and physical activity, or how special-needs daycare programs address quality-of-life issues for disabled children. Following the first four-week field experience, the students have a debriefing tutorial wherein they discuss health determinants in relation to both their field experiences and their selected readings. Over the course of the semester each tutorial group of six students experiences all four agency networks, and in week seven each pair

Donald Wasylenki, Niall Byrne, and Barbara McRobb

of students makes a presentation to their tutorial group, focusing on health determinants.

For the next four weeks each pair of students is placed in a different agency in a different network, and the focus shifts to health promotion strategies. Students use guiding questions to determine how agency activities promote health and/or prevent disability. In week twelve a second debriefing tutorial occurs with selected readings on health promotion. Finally, on completion of the semester, each student submits an essay on health promotion strategies and is given a numerical grade for attendance, participation, and quality of presentation and essay.

———

The third component of the HIC course, Achieving Health in the Community, occupies one half-day per week throughout the second year. Each student selects an agency placement in the community, develops a learning contract, and spends the year studying the interaction of a health problem and a social issue dealt with in the agency placement. At the end of the second year, each student makes a major project presentation to an audience of faculty, peers, hospital staff, and community personnel. Each student also submits a substantial project report. The project presentation outlines the objectives and methods used in the study and presents results and recommendations. Each presentation is twenty minutes in length with additional time for discussion; the reports are 3,000–4,000 words long in a standardized format, and several result in publications in scientific journals each year. This process has been described in detail elsewhere (Wasylenki, Byrne, & McRobb, 1997a).

In order to qualify as a placement, an agency must offer health and/or social services; must be part of a formal or informal network of programs and services; must provide an environment suited to the study of the interaction between a health problem and a social issue; and must provide a field supervisor. During the first HIC session in the second year, students are presented with an extensive list of potential agency placements. Students spend the first six weeks in the course selecting agencies from the list, defining issues, being interviewed by agency staff, and, by mid October, formalizing their placement. If a student is not able to select an agency from the list provided, he/she may propose some other agency in the community which meets the criteria. This selection is described as a "student-initiated choice," and 25–30 percent of placements are "student-initiated." In the first iteration of the second-year HIC, 252 agency placements occurred. Subsequently, the class size has been reduced, and now 177 placements are required. These placements are largely in addition to the roughly 150 agency placements in the second semester of the first year. The HIC course thus involves well over three hundred participating agencies.

Following the selection of an agency, each student develops an individual learning plan (ILP). The ILP follows a set format within which the student outlines project parameters including objectives and activities he or she will undertake. Examples of project themes include homelessness and mental illness, tuberculosis and immigration, and the impact of culture on injury prevention programs. Once the ILP is completed, an HIC coordinator reviews it and the student embarks upon the project. During the months of October and November while the ILP is being developed, two workshops are offered to the students, addressing basic methodological issues in collecting and analyzing data. The first workshop presents qualitative approaches to gathering, analyzing, and presenting information; the second focuses on quantitative approaches. Students are encouraged to incorporate a mixture of qualitative and quantitative methods in their project designs. Other small-group seminars are offered throughout the year to assist with project work, presentation skills, and report writing.

During the second year the student consults with three key individuals. The first is the site coordinator for Achieving Health in the Community. This individual organizes the course for subgroups of students at hospital sites and assists students in making agency selections, developing ILPs, and problem solving as the project unfolds. The second key person is the agency field supervisor. This usually is a senior administrative person who introduces the student and the project to the agency and who helps the student carry out project work both at the agency and beyond as the student explores the community in relation to the topic chosen. The third key person is the resource advisor, a faculty member assigned by the site coordinator to provide the student with expertise, either in methodology or the topic area chosen. This person functions somewhat as a thesis advisor as the student carries out his/her course of study.

In February of the second year, each student submits an ILP progress report indicating the extent to which ILP objectives have been achieved and ILP activities have been carried out. This report also is assessed by the site coordinator and a numerical mark assigned. The overall numerical mark given at the end of the second year is a composite of marks for attendance and participation (assigned by the field supervisor), ILP development, and progress and quality of presentation and report.

Course Management

Over the years, a management structure for HIC has evolved to include faculty members, community agency representatives, and students. Overall responsibility for the course resides with the course director, a physician and full-time faculty member, assisted by a course administrator, another full-time position occupied by a senior administrative staff member with considerable experience in the organization and coordination of physician activities. For the first two components of HIC during the first year, there is a designated HIC facilitator at each of the four teaching hospitals.

For the second component of the course, Promoting Health in the Community, there are four network coordinators linked to the elderly persons' centers, child and family services, drug and alcohol programs, and community health centers. These four coordinators meet regularly as a group. For the third component of HIC (second year), Achieving Health in the Community, there are designated HIC coordinators at each of the four sites of the Faculty of Medicine. These HIC coordinators have major responsibilities with regard to course delivery. Working closely with the course administrator, they compile the agency lists, oversee the agency selection process, support and evaluate ILP development, monitor student progress, assess ILP progress, organize and assess student presentations, and assess student reports.

The HIC course-planning committee is responsible for advising the course director with regard to all aspects of the HIC course. This committee meets monthly for two hours. Membership includes eleven faculty members, four community agency representatives, four students, and the course administrator. Course-planning committee activities include regular review of each of the three course components and consideration of various related issues, such as student assessment, faculty development, student feedback, and proposed modifications to course content and/or delivery. As well, there are four principal subcommittees reporting to the course-planning committee.

In addition to the personnel and committee structure, course management has included a yearly convening of course participants. Initially, this took the form of an agency appreciation night to which all agencies and faculty were invited. In the third year of the course, the agency appreciation night was replaced by a course colloquium. The colloquium involves sixty to seventy representatives of agencies, faculty, and students and is held at the end of or just preceding the beginning of the academic year. The goal is to review the past year's experience and to identify course strengths and weaknesses. In addition to the colloquia, agency participants in the course receive a letter of thanks each year, as well as a certificate signed by the dean of medicine and the course director designating their agency as a Faculty of Medicine teaching site. These certificates appear to be valued by participating agencies. The course administrator also works to facilitate access by community participants to university resources such as libraries and continuing education events. Recently, faculty appointments have been made accessible to agency personnel.

Course Evaluation

Evaluation of the HIC course has been reported elsewhere (Wasylenki, Byrne, & McRobb, 1997b) and has drawn upon a number of sources of information. These include a community questionnaire, student surveys and focus groups, feedback from community agencies, and measures of student performance. Systematic information is available for three cohorts of students. Cohort A entered in the fall of 1992, cohort B in the fall of 1993, and cohort C in the fall of 1994.

Before beginning the HIC course, students complete the community questionnaire. The questionnaire is readministered at the end of the first two course components. For cohort A ($N = 238$), the questionnaire demonstrated significant increases in both positive attitudes and knowledge by the end of the second component. For cohort B ($N = 172$) increases in knowledge were recorded by the end of the second component but positive attitudes showed no change. For cohort C ($N = 146$) very substantial increases in knowledge were recorded by the end of the second component. Attitudes were very positive on first administration and remained very positive, with no change, at year-end.

With regard to the first semester, students in all three cohorts expressed high levels of satisfaction with the home-care field visits. However, students in cohorts B and C rated the public health experience as poor because too much time was spent in public health units and not enough time in the field. One-quarter of students in cohorts A and B stated they did not enjoy the first semester of HIC and 47 percent of students in cohort C rated the first semester as only fair or poor.

For the second semester, students in all three cohorts rated the field visits very positively. Among the four agency networks, drug and alcohol placements and community health centers were somewhat more popular than child and family agencies and elderly persons' centers. The most positive aspect of the second-year course was the agency placement. Three-quarters of students in cohorts A and B rated the agency placement and the agency staff and supervisor as excellent. Three-quarters of respondents stated that, by the end of the course, they were able to evaluate the relationship between a health problem and a social issue for a defined population. Still, one-third of respondents reported that they were dissatisfied with the *overall* second-year experience. Feedback

Donald Wasylenki, Niall Byrne, and Barbara McRobb

from agencies involved in the course, however, has been uniformly positive and enthusiastic.

Fifty patients who participated in the home-care visit sessions were surveyed by phone. The response was overwhelmingly positive. Forty-eight patients thought that the medical student visits were a positive experience, forty-nine believed that the students benefited from the experience, fifty reported that the students behaved appropriately, and forty-one said they would volunteer to participate again.

Roughly 90 percent of agencies involved in the four second-semester networks felt they had provided the students with valuable learning experiences. Almost all have continued to participate throughout the three years. Many agencies interviewed were very eager to participate more in the planning, implementation, and evaluation of the HIC course. Over 90 percent of second-year agency supervisors reported that students in cohorts A and B completed their work in a manner appropriate to the agency's expectations. Ninety-eight percent said that the project was relevant to their agency's mission, and 90 percent reported that the student's project had benefited the agency.

———

Experience with the HIC course indicates that it is possible to organize and maintain community learning experiences for large groups of undergraduate medical students in an urban environment. Course planners have been able to recruit more than 350 agencies as learning sites (Wasylenki, Cohen, & McRobb, 1997c). One of the striking features of the HIC experience has been the extremely positive response to the course by community agencies. As noted, the Home Care Program for Metropolitan Toronto was an immediate and very energetic partner initially, and the six municipal public health units worked hard to create a useful learning experience. All four networks of agencies involved in the second course component have been enthusiastic, and each network has strengthened participation over the four-year period. In the second year, more agency partners are recruited than are ordinarily necessary, and the feedback, as reported, has been very positive. Unfortunately, the medical school has little to give back to participating agencies, as the agencies are voluntary partners in the HIC course. When asked why they continue to participate in the face of general budgetary constraints and lack of fiscal returns, the response continues to be "because we want our doctors to be better!" It appears that agencies participate in the course because they are dissatisfied with the behavior of many doctors with whom they interact; they wish to shape the attitudes and behaviors of physicians in training; they want future doctors to know about their specific programs; and they are eager for doctors to understand the broader context of health care in Toronto.

The strength of the course, from the students' point of view, clearly emerges as the field placements. The home care placements are popular because students encounter persons actually dealing with illness in a community setting. The public health placements were less popular, partially because they were seen as less clinically relevant. The importance of population health is not obvious to students in first-year medical school. More recently, sixteen inner-city schools have been enthusiastic participants. Among the four agency networks in the second semester, the drug and alcohol placements and the community health centers have been most popular. Again, these placements tend to be more clinical than the day centers in the child and family network and the elderly persons' centers. These latter networks have been strengthened with good results. Special-needs daycare placements have been added to normal daycare placements, and elderly persons center placements have been enriched by a variety of other senior support programs. In the second year, the field placements were rated very highly by students as learning experiences, perhaps because of two elements: First, there is much more choice involved, as students are able to select an agency in relation to their own particular interests. Second, the students spend the entire year working in one agency in close collaboration with agency staff, and a strong sense of belonging to the agency appears to develop. Positive relationships with staff evolve, and the students experience high levels of satisfaction. This satisfaction is also manifest in the quality and relevance of the second-year projects, which tend to reflect a sophisticated combination of the students' interests and the agencies' needs.

The most disappointing aspect of the HIC experience for the first three years was the extent of student dissatisfaction. The initial class (cohort A) perceived themselves to be "guinea pigs" in the experiment and saw the HIC course as having replaced highly valued elective time in the curriculum. This led to HIC's being regarded as a below-average course by students in the first cohort. This perception was conveyed to the incoming second cohort, perpetuating the unfavorable view. On closer examination it appears that, whereas the course has been strong in providing interesting field experiences, it has been weaker in structuring a sound theoretical curriculum. This contributes to the students' persistent questioning of the relevance of the course to the practice of medicine. The negative attitudes of some faculty members external to the course toward the concept of community-based learning also contribute to dissatisfaction. More recently, as the course has become a more established aspect of the curriculum and as changes in the health care system have emphasized the importance of community care, attitudes both in students and faculty have become more positive.

Although we were disappointed by student attitudes, we have been satisfied with student performance. Initially, there was some anxiety about how students would behave in patients' homes and in agency placements, especially if they felt resentful about having to be there in the first place. These fears were unwarranted. Agency staff regularly comment upon the professional comportment of students and their obvious interest and enthusiasm. There have been only a few episodes of unprofessional behavior, such as failing to appear for a prearranged appointment, and these have usually been resolved to everyone's satisfaction. We have been especially gratified by the response of patients in the home care program to being visited by the students. As noted, the patients find this an enjoyable experience; they feel it is important to the students' learning and they appear to regard it as an opportunity to contribute to improving health care delivery. With regard to student performance, the presentations, essays, and reports have been of an extremely high caliber. Some students' projects have been featured in the local media, and some have been published and/or submitted for publication in scientific journals. With regard to the impact on student behavior in the final two clinical years, we have begun to receive anecdotes from clinicians to the effect that students in cohorts A and B seem different on the wards, in that there is more sensitivity to a comprehensive array of patient needs for support, and more knowledge about available community resources.

It is our view that the HIC experience is transferable to other medical schools in urban settings. In fact, the University of Western Ontario, in London, has developed a similar course based largely on the Toronto model. It is important, however, that medical school administrators understand the need for considerable resources to support an extensive array of community placements. In addition to a course director (.25 FTE), we have required a full-time course administrator (1 FTE), and a full-time course secretary (1 FTE). Roughly ninety faculty members participate as tutors/lecturers/seminar leaders in our course and between three and four hundred community agencies are involved. We believe that the benefits to students and to the relationship between the medical school and the community are significant and worthwhile, and that the required expenditures represent a very positive investment.

————

We have found that shifting the locus of undergraduate medical education from hospital to community is indeed possible. In particular, we have discovered that large numbers of community agencies are available and interested in providing learning sites. This should be of interest to educators concerned with developing community partnerships. Faculty members, both medical and nonmedical, are enthusiastic about leading tutorials focused on community-centered learning experiences, broad health determinants, and health promotion strategies. Student attitudes toward community-based education are mixed. One-quarter to one-third of students are less than enthusiastic about spending time in community agencies. Student performance, on the other hand, is outstanding, and we have been gratified by the results of student projects in the HIC course. It appears that a solid appreciation of the importance of social and contextual issues is achieved, in spite of some of the students' negative attitudes. The challenge now is to extend this example into the clerkship component of undergraduate education in order to enhance the initial knowledge and skills developed in our preclerkship course.

Donald Wasylenki, Niall Byrne, and Barbara McRobb

EDWARD J. ECKENFELS

The Case for Keeping
Community Service Voluntary

Narratives from the Rush Community Service Initiatives Program

The Rush Community Service Initiatives Program (RCSIP) is a thriving, self-perpetuating network consisting of a broad spectrum of community service programs that match student initiative and enthusiasm with the social and health needs of prescribed segments of the Chicago population (Eckenfels, 1993; Eckenfels, 1997; Eckenfels, Baier, Turner-Roan, & Sanchez, 1994). The primary aim of the program is to enhance the personal learning and development of medical students in preparation for meeting the health needs of a changing society by providing health and social services to poor and disadvantaged communities.

The impetus for this venture came from a small group of students who voiced a concern that something vital was missing in their education, something that went beyond the scientific underpinnings, the clinical competency, and the technical skills that constituted the traditional, formal medical school curriculum. What they felt was being left out was an affirmation of the core values that motivated them to become physicians in the first place, namely, the moral consciousness, the social responsibility, the idealism that they believed were the foundation of the medical profession.

It had become evident to them that compassion, sensitivity, and cultural awareness didn't fit into the biomedical construct. In addition, they were constantly told that there was simply too much knowledge and technique to learn, too many technical and scientific advances to master, and too much information to absorb. Moreover, the inside dopesters — upperclassmates who had learned to work the system (see Berger, 1963) — had made it patently clear that everything that really matters, everything that was worthwhile, took place outside the formal structure in what Hafferty calls "the hidden curriculum," where the emphasis was on finding a specialty and a set of procedures to provide a good life and successful career (Hafferty & Franks, 1994). It wasn't long, however, before this group of vociferous students found that many of their own classmates had similar concerns; they too shared a sense of isolation and constriction by having the vast majority of their education take place within or under the aegis of the academic health center. For them, the real world, the world that they hoped to practice in, was outside this tertiary care setting.

All of this was made known to me in a course I taught on community health and social medicine during the spring quarter of their first year in 1989. My primary course objective was simply to get the students outside the walls of the academic health center and into the vast cultural diversity of Chicago. Small groups of students (no more than six) were assigned three different site visits to neighborhood health centers, public health agencies, HMOs, and the like, which were followed, two days later, by small-group discussions facilitated by a clinician and one other faculty member. The students were given a checklist of things to look for (e.g., staff morale, quality of services offered, client satisfaction) to guide them in summarizing their experiences. The discussions that followed the site visits were intense and emotional. The students talked openly and freely about the poor and underserved communities they had visited, the quality of care delivered in the neighborhood clinics, and the sociocultural barriers to medical services they had observed. My colleagues and I learned that a large number of them were also concerned that medicine was forsaking its societal responsibility by giving in to market demands as the primary force in shaping health care policy. Many of them embraced the belief that health care was a right, not a business. In addition, a common theme among the discussion groups was the need for reaffirmation of their values and beliefs through some form of collective social action.

At the completion of the course, a number of students approached me to tell me that this simple course, with its limited time allotment (only twenty-four hours) and placement in the same quarter as neuroscience and microbiology, was their only exposure to what they thought was essential to maintaining their sense of purpose in the pursuit of their career goals. They wanted more. Although I was quite flattered and somewhat astonished, I pointed out that there was no room in the already overcrowded schedule to add more time for these activities, and it was too late to try to make any changes in the curriculum. (They had no idea of the obstacles involved in getting a curriculum committee to even consider change, let alone add more time for a subject like this.) They concluded that if more community experiences couldn't be added to the formal curriculum, they would arrange them on their own as an extracurricular activity. I listed a number of concerns they would have to deal with — first, and foremost, finding sites that could use their services, and, if they were to be involved in any kind

Edward J. Eckenfels

of health care, they would need physician mentors, medical supplies and drugs, and malpractice insurance, to mention a few basic considerations. One by one, they solved these problems. They found a clinic that could use their help, recruited faculty members who wanted to join them, found drug company representatives who were willing to donate samples, and, with the aid of the medical center legal council, were able to resolve the insurance issue through a careful reading of the Good Samaritan Act in Illinois and the institution's coverage of them as members of Rush.

These efforts, which had begun in 1989 and were activated in 1990, served as the genesis for the establishment of RCSIP as an actual entity. In 1991 the core group of student organizers and I (as their unofficial faculty advisor) devised an organizational structure with goals, objectives, and a mission statement. In 1991 the program designers agreed that, to be successful in meeting these goals, RCSIP had to (1) be student-run, (2) be voluntary, (3) provide continuity of service, and (4) demonstrate its efficacy through systematic evaluation. In addition, programs were to be broad in scope, range across the life cycle, and encompass populations representative of Chicago's vast cultural, ethnic, and racial mix. An office was set up in the Department of Preventive Medicine which housed a director, assistant director, and program assistant. Since its inception, RCSIP has instituted eighteen different initiatives that include participation in four free clinics, numerous counseling and educational programs, and a range of activities from serving as Big Sibs to infants and children who are HIV-seropositive to the functional assessment of the elderly. During this period, funding was acquired from the Frye Foundation, AT&T, the Rockefeller Foundation, the Pew Charitable Trusts, the Robert Wood Johnson Foundation, and the Chicago Northern Trust. Two years ago, RCSIP was made a permanent program of the medical center.

Reflection on this past decade leads me to believe that the most significant aspect of RCSIP, the sustaining ingredient, the raison d'être, has been the students' awareness that this was *their* opportunity to act passionately on what they believed in, to give freely of themselves in a cause that was worthwhile and of their *own making*. They advocated the notion that *volunteerism* was the essential element for giving meaning to their actions. They adopted the position that being outside the constraints of the formal structure allows them to do things entirely on their own, thus providing the real conditions for altruism, duty, and authentic development (AAMC, 1998). Likewise, from its beginning, participation in RCSIP offered these students an outlet for overcoming their frustrations and sense of isolation. In RCSIP they found a community of peers who not only shared some of the same values but openly expressed them. Furthermore, the obstacles encountered in the creation of RCSIP (including the medical school's concern regarding level of competence, safety issues, etc.) presented them with the opportunity to use creative solutions to meet these challenges. They formulated strategies and employed them effectively. Adversity broadened their perspective and spurred them on. In short, RCSIP fostered a true maturation process.

In my effort to understand the effect on these young people of their participation in these voluntary community service projects, I have become more and more aware that their efforts affect them very deeply. Their personal involvement outside the academic health center seems to give special meaning to their sense of purpose — why they are here in the first place — regardless of the impediments and obstacles they encounter in the course of their traditional medical training and professional socialization. As Coles (1993) observed, "Service is a means of putting to use what we have learned — to connect moral ideals to the lived life" (p. xxiii). The effect that I have observed on many of our students is profound. They see and feel the world differently. In some cases their experience is a powerful reinforcement of what they already believe. For others it is an awakening of a social conscience. At the very least, it is an experience that stands out as an act of personal volition and commitment.

Narratives as a Window to the Heart

I can't think of a better way to capture the meaning of these voluntary community service experiences than in the students' own words. Here are a few examples of what I mean.

Peter, who is active in three programs, was asked why he was willing to become a "big sib" to a child who is HIV-seropositive. He answered by first showing us a photo of Rudy, his "little pal." Without hesitating, he began to relate the history of his relationship with his friend. The child had been adopted when he was still an infant. The home of the adopting parents, while comfortable, was far from ideal. The father had bouts of alcoholism, an older brother deeply resented the boy, and the mother was overindulgent in her attempt to show her love for this "forsaken child." While taking great care to protect the identity of the boy, Peter vividly described his relationship with Rudy, the places they visited (the zoo, museums), the limits he set (there was only so much dinosaur paraphernalia he could afford), and the significant role he was playing in the boy's life (Rudy wished Peter were his "real" brother). When asked what all of this meant to him personally, Peter, who is going to be a pediatrician, replied, "I love kids. Rudy has AIDS; he is going to die. I want to remain human and loving when I have to deal with the death of a child. It may seem selfish, but I simply can't wait until I am a full-fledged doctor. I know I have so much to gain from him. I hope I can give something in return."

Amy, a first-year medical student, had recently become involved in the in-service training of five local-community asthma workers at Henry Horner, a Chicago Housing Authority project next to the United Center where the Bulls play basketball. She relayed the following story about her initial experience in the training session:

> This experience had a profound effect on me. I think it changed my life. Actually, I don't know how to describe it. Here were these five women. Some of them had spent their entire lives in Horner. All of them had children. One had seven. But they are such loving mothers — they are so considerate. They are so wise. They are angry with the insensitivity of society toward them (they have every right to be) — lack of health care, insensitive doctors, all that stuff. But they weren't hostile toward us! In fact they were kind and considerate. They were like our teachers, explaining things to us, describing what life is like in the projects. When I got home, I called my mother. I told her I thought I knew something about how poor people survive in the projects, but I knew nothing. They are loving mothers who need a chance. How fortunate we are. How fortunate I am to get to know them. I hope I can help them in some way.

Craig, another student, had to deal with a number of setbacks and dead ends in trying to establish a new program for the homeless. It was quite an education for him, having been stonewalled by both public and private agencies. He was misled and, in one case, actually lied to about a potential site. But, despite all the frustrations and obstacles, he remained committed to his goal of starting a free clinic at a homeless shelter. His perseverance finally paid off when he hooked up with a family doctor who provides medical services at a homeless shelter. Since his initial encounter with the shelter, Craig has taken with him some nursing students who are also interested in community service and the health of the homeless. This is his answer to why he is concerned with the plight of the homeless:

> No one really cares about the homeless any more. In fact, people not only have become immune to them — they despise them! They see them as cra-zies, druggies, terrorizers, nuts. A lot of this is true, in one sense. But they are human beings in need. You would have to be an idiot to believe that simply providing limited medical care is the answer to their problems. But, for ex-ample, when I was there last Tuesday night, and after we had worked up all

of the patients — lots of respiratory problems and TB, the shelter staff has tested positive — you have to walk through this big open bay with all of these men [there is a separate room for the women] sleeping on cots. And you hear them snoring, and coughing, and breathing heavily. And you know that they are just like you, they are living, breathing, human beings. No more and no less, and they deserve to be treated as such.

An especially revealing indication of the effect of these community service experiences can be found in the open-ended responses from our study of patients' perceptions of quality of care and students' assessments of learning and development in the student-run prenatal clinic. This study was directed by Michelle Bardack, M.D., a fourth-year medical student at that time, and one of the principal founders of the prenatal service at Saint Basil's Free People's Clinic on Chicago's southwest side. In the time allotted — an eight-week elective course — medical records were analyzed and in-depth interviews were conducted with fifteen of the thirty clinic patients and eleven of the thirteen students who administered the prenatal care. The medical records showed that the patients received excellent prenatal care resulting in healthy babies and normal deliveries. Fourteen of the fifteen respondents rated the quality of care the best they had ever received and characterized the students as personable, sensitive, knowledgeable, and deeply caring.

Again, here are some typical responses about how volunteering in the clinic influenced career choices:

[At the clinic] I realized I wanted to become, and could become, an independent family practitioner with an active obstetrical practice, and so I looked into family practice residencies that offered a strong OB experience.

The clinic experience was extremely important to my residency decision, as I quickly learned that doing OB outside the tertiary care center was indeed very different. It was a great experience to see community OB (I loved it) whereas my hospital clerkship almost turned me off.

Usually in my hospital clerkships I learned what kind of doctor I do not want to be; at Saint Basil's I was able to learn what kind of doctor I wanted to be — it solidified my ideas to look for a primary care residency.

When asked what they gained from their participation at the clinic, all of them indicated the experience was a highly positive and beneficial one. However, their personal comments provide a real sense of the true development that has been facilitated and sustained in this nurturing and compassionate setting.

Edward J. Eckenfels

They remarked that they "don't get exposed to a continuity care experience in school, or to such a level of responsibility"; that "[the clinic] was unlike any other experience I had in medical school; learning to relate to people of other cultures and backgrounds was as important as the academic experience"; that "this hands-on experience exposed me to a whole different perspective on health care issues — those outside the hospital — I found myself and my patient sometimes overwhelmed when trying to solve some of the social problems my patient faced."

In addition, students' exposure to the patients' "human" problems had a lasting effect. One student told of a patient who needed an applicator for her medicine but whose public aid care would not cover it: "I kept telling her to purchase one at her local pharmacy, and she kept returning to the clinic sick and without having taken the medicine. She was still sick and I was frustrated. Finally it came out that she didn't have even the few dollars necessary to purchase the applicator." Another student told of a pregnant nineteen-year-old who worked at McDonald's to support her other child and her husband: the smell made her so nauseated that she rarely ate enough. Her husband was becoming abusive and she wanted to leave, but with such a low-paying job, with one child and one on the way, she felt she had no other options.

> I picked her [the patient] up at her house, and for the first time saw how she lived — with her grandmother and multiple relatives. There was very little heat in the middle of the winter, in a very small apartment, with very little furniture, and one bed for a family of four.

This final commentary provides a good summary of the meaning of the "total experience" for these students:

> For the first time I became aware of the existence of the working poor. I never would have gotten such a sense of community had I remained at the tertiary care hospital for four years; the experience reminded me of the reasons I came to medical school — for service to the community and to develop relationships that help people improve their lives.

Volunteerism as a Source of Authenticity

Authenticity is a contemporary moral ideal. It is not hedonism or self-centered individualism. The root of this kind of authenticity is, to use Charles Taylor's (1991) description, like an inner voice telling us the right thing to do, "something we have to attain to be true and full human beings" (p. 26). This is exactly the ideal I have witnessed in students who view medicine as a calling — a higher calling — in which their lives would not be fulfilled without it. The practice of medicine, for them, is more than the knowledge and skills of a competent practitioner. They look for authenticity in their learning and development in keeping with the higher moral good that attracted them to medicine in the first place.

It should be evident by now from what I have argued in this essay that the *voluntary, student-generated* aspects of RCSIP provide the ideal milieu for promoting authenticity. Seifer and others (1996) take exception to this view. They state that although we "encourage and support volunteerism . . . the learning that occurs . . . is not *structured* [emphasis mine] and may be quite accidental" (p. 275). In another paper, Seifer, Mutha, and Connors (1996) suggest that service learning "linked to specific course-based learning objectives has a greater impact on students than do elective or voluntary experiences" (p. 36). Is it really possible to distinguish between "service" and "learning?" Where does the service end and the learning begin, and vice versa? On what basis do they conclude that the learning that takes place in "voluntary" programs is "accidental"? Many of the most important lessons we learn in life — be they values and beliefs or factual knowledge — are accidental, that is, not based on prearranged and carefully prescribed duties and assignments. One of the most human and essential sources of satisfaction in life comes from dealing with uncertainty — an activity which, incidentally, is at the core of being a physician. Although I am certain that the students who participate in prearranged and required experiences in community settings benefit from them, I find no basis to support the assumption that "course-based learning objectives [have] a greater impact on the students."

The reference here, of course, is to the *program designers'* learning objectives. *They* determine if the experience was successful (i.e., meaningful, educational, developmental) based on whether or not the participants met *their* stated aims. Do those learning objectives include altruism, advocacy, and other forms of moral development, and, if so, how are they measured? I have seen the variety and complexity of questionnaires, scales, and other assessment tools program designers have developed, and, like most bureaucracies, such means of assessment can become an iron cage. As Goulet (1971) notes, to reduce the totality of these experiences "to that mere portion of reality which is measurable is to deprive life of its specificity and to falsify reality itself" (p. 208).

It is the very *unmediated* nature of RCSIP that makes it such a powerful experience. Too much structure, especially in consciousness-raising exercises like

Edward J. Eckenfels

providing community service, prevents the participants from developing freely (Claxton, 1997). Furthermore, RCSIP promotes active *problem solving*; that is, the participants have to create their own structure that fits with their other demands (academic and personal) and, at the same time, keep the programs running effectively.

The spinoffs from such responsibilities include acquiring the administrative and interpersonal skills needed for program development, such as scheduling, orientation, evaluation, training, and the like. Moreover, the very act of being in charge of providing service requires critical reasoning, empathy, and a nonjudgmental spirit. The issues at stake pertain to the community, its members, and the social ills that influence the well-being of everyone involved. By immersing themselves in real-world settings that are not mediated by external structural constraints (i.e., those not of their own making), the students are faced with social and political situations that challenge conventional notions of community development. These experiences have a profound effect on the participants without teaching them a single fact. The ethical issues confronting students participating in voluntary community service programs include poverty, racism, discrimination, and the decline of public trust.

Voluntary service — no strings attached — allows the provider to experience the meaning of *altruism*, that rare human quality that gives true meaning to life. Moreover, the *personal* reflections that come from such acts (frequently in informal, nonscheduled discussions with other participants, close friends, or family members) allows the volunteer to *examine* what it means — the most important lessons to be learned from such encounters. To be fully yourself without regard to others is self-defeating. But to get what you want out of life in a way that contributes to society is the kind of authenticity I see students in RCSIP striving for. It allows them to feel the satisfaction of making a contribution by giving freely of themselves and, at the same time, allows others to get more out of their lives as well. As Taylor (1991) would say, they seek "horizons of significance" and find them on their own.

LUCY WOLF TUTON

CLAUDIA H. SIEGEL

TIMOTHY B. CAMPBELL

Bridging the Gaps

Community Health Internship Program

A Case Study in the Professional Development of Medical Students

As our scientific and technological knowledge has expanded, success in medical care has often been measured through new medical advances, new genes discovered, or medical technology invented. Medical science has assisted in saving the youngest life and extending the oldest, developing therapies for debilitating and once incurable conditions, and uncovering information about the human body and disease processes that was previously unknown. These developments have helped to shape a paradigm of medical science and a system of health care that focuses on individual diseases and seeks out new technology, biochemistry, microbiology, and pharmacology to cure the sicknesses we see around us. Our process of medical education has also been built upon this view, generating large numbers of practitioners who are scientifically adept, disease oriented, and technologically inclined.

Yet as our body of scientific knowledge has grown, we have come to realize that, though many academic health centers lie within or near economically deprived neighborhoods, their presence has had limited effect in changing the awful realities that influence community life and health. For example, sustaining the life of a two-pound premature infant does not solve the problem of infant mortality in the United States, which ranked twenty-fifth among industrialized nations in 1993 (United States Department of Health and Human Services, 1997). Indeed, in communities surrounding some prestigious academic health centers, many births occur without the mothers' receiving adequate, if any, prenatal care. These births are ultimately "high risk" because of factors that lie outside the control of the medical science which enables the hospital and its physicians to sustain these small lives.

The challenge of medical professional development is that we must educate our students in both the technology and the humanity of health care delivery. It is our responsibility to produce health care professionals whose technical competencies are above question. They must also have the attitudes, knowledge, and skills to understand and influence the environmental and community factors affecting health; to deliver culturally competent care grounded in health promotion and disease prevention; and to act as advocates for those who need care in a system that is increasingly parsimonious in its use of available resources. These attitudes and skills are grounded in a broader view of health care than one circumscribed by technology, genetics, and pharmacology. This broader view encompasses the values of compassion, communication, tolerance, and accountability, values that can be easily obscured by considerations of the "bottom line," the latest pharmacological or genetic solutions to patients' problems, and the generally disjointed organization of health care delivery. Reinvigorating medical professional training with this broader view requires that we give our students more diverse experiences outside of traditional medical academic environments, and that we add the perspective of community to that of the academic health center. The community exposes students to circumstances that contribute to the wellness or illness of their future patients, and compels students to respond constructively to the larger human and social context in which health professionals function.

Bridging the Gaps (BTG) provides medical and other health and social service professional students with an intensive health-related community service experience in partnership with community organizations. The program originated at one medical school, where faculty with experience and interest in community health asked colleagues at another school if they were interested in joining the program. One by one additional academic health centers joined. The program started with eighteen medical students. In 1998, the program included 165 students from multiple disciplines in Philadelphia, 14 at the University of Pittsburgh, and 10 at Lake Erie College of Osteopathic Medicine.

The program relies heavily on community expertise and guidance, bringing together institutional and community resources to accomplish the program's multiple objectives. The program consists of on-site community experiences combined with didactic skill-building sessions. The disciplines involved in the program over the years have included medicine, nursing, social work, dentistry, pharmacy, physical therapy, occupational therapy, physician assisting, public health, creative arts therapy, and law.

Bridging the Gaps is an elective program. Some of the institutions give credit for the experience. The medical students participate between their first and second years. Students from other disciplines are at different levels depending on their discipline. For the community-based portion of the experience, students are matched with community placement sites based on student interest and community need. Whenever possible, students are placed in interdisciplinary teams. The program begins in June and continues for seven weeks. Each team or student defines a site-related project with assistance from community preceptors as well as preceptors from the academic institutions. The academic preceptor serves as a resource and/or role model for the student experience. Academic preceptors meet regularly with their students to discuss work at the community site. They also review the student's weekly journal, final paper, and poster. Perhaps the most important role of the academic preceptors is in providing input into project development and implementation. The community preceptor serves as a site mentor for the student and an advocate for the community. The community preceptor also evaluates the student's work and its impact on his/her agency or program.

Collaborating community agencies and organizations include homeless shelters, summer camps, public housing developments, substance abuse treatment facilities, and community health clinics, among others. Students develop projects that assist their community organizations in responding to health-related needs. Projects may involve community health assessment, health promotion and outreach activities, research into specific community health problems, and planning, organizing, and implementing health education programs. In the 1998 program year, the majority of the 189 student participants reported dealing with a variety of community health issues at least once, including diet and nutrition, exercise, communication, cardiovascular risk, substance abuse, HIV/AIDS, and personal hygiene. Among the other issues students encountered were culture-specific health beliefs and practices, child care, chronic illness, insurance and social service, and sexual questions and issues (Bridging the Gaps Network, 1998). BTG monitors the issues encountered by students through a measurement instrument which students complete on a daily basis (see discussion of accountability below).

BTG shares program progress with the broader public health and social service communities through an annual fall symposium, an annual "health action report" which documents the work of the program, and presentations at national meetings. It is administered by representatives from seven of Pennsylvania's eight academic health centers (Lake Erie College of Osteopathic Medicine (LECOM), MCP Hahnemann University, Philadelphia College of Osteopathic Medicine, Temple University, Thomas Jefferson University, the University of Pennsylvania, and the University of Pittsburgh). The five institutions in Philadelphia join together to develop and implement a variety of program elements, including curriculum, evaluation, and fundraising. Each institution also implements its own component program in response to the needs of the institution and its surrounding community. The programs at LECOM and the University of Pittsburgh revolve around community health needs in Erie and Pittsburgh, respectively. All of the programs participate in the annual symposium in Philadelphia and are profiled in the annual report.

———

BTG is grounded in collaboration. This value guides relationships among academic health centers, between health and social service disciplines, and between academic health centers and communities. Each aspect of the program offers an opportunity to illustrate to students the personal and professional importance of collaboration and of forming mutually beneficial relationships based on trust and respect.

From the first day of the program students understand that they are entering an established network based on collaboration. This network provides support, but also demands accountability. Over the course of the program, students come to understand that, in their professional role, the development of ongoing collaborative relationships will be the key to effective service provision.

For many students, entry into a working relationship in an underserved community is initially unfamiliar and sometimes unsettling. However, students are supported by the collaboration that has preceded them. Each institution's program coordinators have worked to develop relationships with the community over time based on a proven track record of cooperation and mutual benefit.[1] Building on these relationships, each class of students constructs their own personal connections with the community and, as the summer progresses, the individual student's perspective changes from "me" and "them," to "us." The relationships formed in the community also enable students to recognize and change their own preconceived notions about underserved populations as well as about other health disciplines. These changes are frequently noted by both students and preceptors in their evaluations of BTG.

Over the course of the program, students learn the central role of trust in collaborative relationships at many different levels. Students must form reciprocal trusting relationships with their colleagues, their preceptors, and those whom they serve. In the context of the community, they rapidly learn that to accomplish collaborative goals, everyone's contribution to a project must be respected and valued. As students learn the skill of collaborating, mutual respect and trust alter their views of once unfamiliar terrain. A 1996 medical student–participant observed about his project environment, "Although Abbottsford [a low-income housing development] may not be as pretty, I feel a greater sense of togetherness than I have ever felt in my own hometown, which is a suburb in New Jersey" (Bridging the Gaps: Philadelphia Community Health Internship Program, 1996, p. 11).

Collaboration also results in student appreciation of a community's expertise, its voice, and its strengths. Ultimately this encourages students to move away from a deficit model of underserved communities and their individual members. Student evaluations of the program have commented on this aspect of their BTG experiences as well, noting that the contribution of community members to student education often surpasses what students bring to the community, particularly in lessons about life and the meaning of hardship and endurance.

———

Significant professional development takes place in the community setting, but on-site experiences are notably enhanced by BTG's didactic curriculum. This curriculum includes an orientation designed to familiarize students with each other as well as with community resources, concepts of community, population diversity, and safety. The orientation utilizes the skills of academic and community personnel. Over the program's seven weeks, students are given an overview of health beliefs, health literacy, safety net issues, innovative health education techniques, violence and its social repercussions, and health insurance and its effect on access to care. In addition to presentations and large-group discussions, small-group sessions are facilitated by community and academic preceptors. Students are encouraged to relate curriculum content to their community experiences. Overall, the didactic curriculum increases student competency to understand a patient or client population on their own terms and to work across cultures, social classes, and educational backgrounds. The combination of the didactic curriculum and the community-based experience brings home to students the importance of providing services that incorporate community resources. Perhaps most important, the didactic curriculum teaches students how to learn from those they serve. The didactic curriculum is revised on an annual basis in response to student evaluations to assure its relevance to students and community. In addition, community preceptor input helps to keep the curriculum current and responsive to the dynamics of community life.

On-site experiences and the didactic curriculum validate the community's stature as a learning resource and an expert in its own milieu. Community members and agency personnel serve as teachers and mentors in the didactic part of the program so that formal mentoring relationships between community and student are established at the outset of the BTG experience. Students learn that the one-sided authority of doctor-patient communication in a health care setting becomes reversed in a community setting. As one student put it, "I think the most important thing I've learned is that if you want to improve the health and fitness of a community, you have to start by giving them what they need and want — not what *you* think they need" (Bridging the Gaps: Philadelphia Community Health Internship Program, 1997, p. 23).

The reciprocal nature of human communication in any service context is a central focus of the program's didactic and experiential curriculum. Student evaluations of their experiences have noted the importance of respectful communication and the difference it made in the community's perceptions of health care professionals. Here are three students' impressions:

Time and time again our clients complained that they were treated like unwelcome, subhuman burdens at local hospitals. On occasions when we provided health care services, it was amazing how grateful our patients were, not so much for the care, which was very basic and usually inadequate, but simply for being treated with dignity and respect. (Bridging the Gaps: Philadelphia Community Health Internship Program, 1997, p. 37)

Not only did we achieve our goal of educating the children about their health, but just from our presence, we helped to change the attitudes of some community members toward health professionals. (Bridging the Gaps: Philadelphia Community Health Internship Program, 1996, p. 30)

It seems that the widest gaps are those that are created in our own minds and in the minds of those whom we would serve. We cannot escape our histories and legacies, but only press on and include patient diplomacy in our outreach efforts, and remember that we are privileged to be able to serve. (Bridging the Gaps: Philadelphia Community Health Internship Program, 1997, p. 52)

Through the program's evaluation process, students learn that they are accountable to their clients, their sites, the program, and the grantmakers who have invested in them. The program creates a context in which students become an important part of a community, and as such they need to take responsibility for what they are accomplishing within the community.

The evaluation process uses both qualitative and quantitative measures to evaluate student and program performance. Students are required to maintain individual journals that are reviewed by program coordinators and academic preceptors at each institution. They are also required to complete a brief questionnaire for each day they are in the community. The questionnaire gathers information on students' activities, the population(s) they encountered, and the community health issues they dealt with. At the conclusion of the program, these data are aggregated to provide communities, students, and funders an overall profile of the year's program. Students also write an individual final paper, and, in addition, develop a project poster with the other members of their team. Student posters are displayed at the annual program symposium in a context of dialogue with community representatives, public health officials, agency personnel, grantmakers, and university faculty and staff. The symposium also brings home the collaborative emphasis of the program because it offers an opportunity for networking among the diverse agencies, organizations, and individuals working on public health issues.

Students' multiple and varied presentations of their project's daily activities, methods, meaning, and goals help them to see the transformation of the project from beginning to end, and frequently help them to see the transformation in themselves, as health professionals and as people. One student wrote,

> I never thought I had so many preconceived notions regarding people. I know it sounds like a cliché to say you should never make assumptions about other people based on their appearances or on what you think someone from a particular background is like, but that is just what I got out of the Bridging the Gaps program. (Bridging the Gaps: Philadelphia Community Health Internship Program, 1997, p. 46)

An annual program report, which is distributed locally, regionally, and nationally, describes the activities of the program year, including individual descriptions of each student project. From all of these activities, students gain an understanding of the larger context in which their work takes place. Perhaps most important, they learn they are accountable to share what they have been doing, so that others can learn from their successes and failures.

BTG is only one influence among many in the professional development of medical students. As a learning experience, it has the potential of building awareness of the characteristics and skills that make providers effective for *all* populations.

Students find that what they are taught in the classroom is only part of the equation. This realization is a powerful ally in the effort to develop physicians who see health in a broader context:

> I . . . learned of the gaps in the provision of health care—it is not enough to provide accessible, cost-effective, quality health care; the population for whom it is intended must have faith in its quality, and must feel that their health is the primary concern of that provider, that there are no ulterior mo-

tives involved and that the providers are sensitive to and knowledgeable about their lifestyle and culture. (G. Taylor, personal communication, August, 1996)

Some students leave the program with the realization that their future as health care professionals will involve advocacy as well as patient care. One student wrote that "this experience has strengthened my resolve to be a patient advocate as well as shown me a new avenue in which to accomplish this goal" (Bridging the Gaps: Philadelphia Community Health Internship Program, 1996, p. 13). In other cases, students have cited the pivotal role of their community collaboration in influencing their decisions about their professional futures: "On a personal and professional level this internship meant a great deal to me. . . . After this experience, I have decided on a career in public health and preventive medicine, possibly with a focus in gynecology and/or women's health" (S. S. Yom, personal communication, August, 1996).

––––––––

As this chapter illustrates, the BTG experience is designed to reflect the values of collaboration, communication, tolerance, and accountability. Our program strives to impart to students a conception of the health care professional as community partner. We firmly believe that this is best done in an experiential way. Needless to say, BTG does not have an equal impact on every student, and some students may feel that it has limited relevance to their professional development.

However, in the many cases where the program succeeds, it can have a long-term impact, both on professionals and on the community. In the words of an alumnus:

The Children's Hospital of Philadelphia (CHOP), where I am currently a second-year resident, serves many children from the community of West Philadelphia, and my primary care clinic is mainly comprised of children from this neighborhood. My experience in Bridging the Gaps has given me invaluable insight into this community that I now serve as a practitioner. . . . I have found that my Bridging the Gaps experience has been invaluable in my interactions with patients and their families as I advance in my training. . . . It is an experience that I continue to learn from even though I have long since finished my internship. (L. K. Lee, personal communication, April 15, 1998)

And in the words of the community:

I have watched these medical students move from wide-eyed students to impassioned young physicians with a strong sense of the complexities of their patients' needs. I have been very proud to be a part of this transition in these young healers, and very proud to be a part of the program which gives them this opportunity. (T. DeFazio, personal communication, October 28, 1998)

As teachers and professionals, we know that no single educational experience determines a student's professional development, but we believe that an experience that highlights the values of compassion, communication, tolerance, and accountability can have as great an impact as a basic science course or a clinical rotation.

NOTES

1. All institutions participating in BTG have adopted the model statement of the program, which clearly articulates the values of cooperation and mutual benefit. The BTG model requires that academic health institutions:

identify an underserved community with whom they hope to collaborate and build service-linked partnerships;

provide continuity of contact between students and faculty at the academic health institution, and the identified community and its organizations and agencies;

develop and integrate didactic and skill-building components for students, based on the assumption that there is a set of skills necessary to provide care to underserved populations;

ensure that supervision is provided by both academic and community preceptors;

regularly evaluate the program by eliciting and incorporating input from participating community and agency personnel, students, faculty, and the people served by the program; and

inform the community of the progress of the program through a public forum and an annual report.

ACKNOWLEDGEMENTS

We gratefully acknowledge former Bridging the Gaps program coordinators who also contributed to the development and implementation of the Bridging the Gaps program: Dave Davison, Sylvia Fields, Euncie D. Franklin, Dee Bill-Harvey, Maureen M. Hourigan, Mary Anne Johnston, Cynthia Livingston, Janice Nevin, Ana Núñez, Carol Melvin Pate, Harriet L. Rubenstein, Robyn Weyand, Nancy Zabaga.

The Bridging the Gaps Network consisted of Mary Ellen Bradley, MCP Hahnemann University; Eddy Bresnitz, Hahnemann University; Carol Cochran, Temple University; Kenneth Epstein, Thomas Jefferson University; Mira Gohel, Thomas Jefferson University; Jeane Ann Grisso, University of Pennsylvania; Valerie Hamaday, Philadelphia College of Osteopathic Medicine; Melissa Herring, Philadelphia College of Osteopathic Medicine; Maria Hervada-Page, Thomas Jefferson University; Marian Laurenzi-Lasky, MCP Hahnemann University; Inyanga Mack, Temple University; Eugene Mochan, Philadelphia College of Osteopathic Medicine; Bonnie O'Connor, MCP Hahnemann University; Susan Rattner,

Thomas Jefferson University; Anthony L. Rostain, University of Pennsylvania; Donald F. Schwarz, University of Pennsylvania; Vincent Zarro, M., MCP Hahnemann University; Jane A. Comi, Lake Erie College of Osteopathic Medicine; Robert E. Evans, Lake Erie College of Osteopathic Medicine; Joyce Holl, University of Pittsburgh; and Thomas O'Toole, University of Pittsburgh

JANET BICKEL

Afterword

"Good Seeds": Growing the Physicians We Need

What does a commitment to improving the professional development of medical students look like? And how can we more positively influence students to become activists on behalf of their patients and communities? Our authors offer a wealth of insights, critiques, and examples. Instead of summarizing these, this concluding chapter zeros in on the most urgent challenges and opportunities at the intersection of professional development and social consciousness.

In their chapter found here, Coulehan and Williams describe entering medical students as "good seeds" too often exposed to "defoliants" and deprived of nourishment. How can we better nourish students' sprouts of social consciousness? Should medical educators give the same emphasis to students' developing professional attitudes and values as they do to the acquisition of biomedical knowledge? As funding for medical education evaporates, forcing reconsideration of priorities, what can be done to prepare physicians who, even in the face of financial disincentives, will remain committed patient advocates and serve the communities most in need?

———

Medical education is a heavily nested system, with medical students operating within a microsystem of residents and multiple tiers and types of faculty, plus patients, nurses, and other health care providers. This microsystem sits within a macrosystem of the academic medical center and university administrators whose worlds are shaped by federal legislation, state budgets, insurance companies, and diverse other chaotic forces (Christakis, 1996). At this juncture, a number of these forces are having the uniformly destabilizing effect of pitting the clock against the needs of individuals throughout the "nest" — patients, students, faculty, department heads. As Christakis and Feudtner (1997) observe, "The healing touch in major medical centers rarely lingers — where are students to learn about building long-term relationships with patients, as most of their encounters with patients and what they witness of patient-physician relationships are 'mere temporary matters,' lacking the deeper human connection that can be the most rewarding aspect of medicine?" (p. 739). This "enforced expediency" has many deleterious consequences for the professional development of physicians. Empathy takes time, but with so little opportunity to connect with patients, how are students to develop this essential perspective? With attending physicians stretched so thin, where are students' sources of inspiration to become active in improving the care their patients receive?

A recent study of attending physicians found that fewer than 42 percent were considered excellent role models by the house staff (Wright et al., 1998). Skeff and Mutha (1998) comment that "unless institutions provide time for a greater number of faculty members to demonstrate their professional roles effectively . . . institutional leaders may have to accept that fewer than half of their teachers will be perceived as effective role models by those they teach" (p. 2017). A recent study of ward teams produced even more troubling results. Attending physicians identified three categories of problematic behaviors in residents and students: showing disrespect for patients, cutting corners, and outright hostility toward patients (Burack et al., 1999). But attendings rarely responded to these behaviors. When they did, they relied on passive nonverbal cues such as rigid posture, on humor, or on medicalization of interpersonal issues; one attending explained that hostility would impede getting good information from patients (p. 52). This study is alarming evidence of faculty detachment from many of the needs of both patients and students.

We all understand the human nature illustrated by the famous faculty quote: "My fellows, our residents, the students." But a result of this distancing is that students are "left to devise answers to fundamental questions, for themselves and by themselves. Who am I? A person, or merely a succession of graduated roles?" (Christakis & Feudtner, 1997, p. 743). Listen to a medical student's own words written as a poem and lament: "My parents are now / white-coated lecturers bringing / simultaneous information . . . / photos of people who you want to cry about so you laugh . . . / I've learned to live on promises / of a better day next week, next year / when Thursday comes, I may forget why I came" (Wong, 1999). Wagoner's chapter here dissects the vicissitudes of this "identity purgatory" and suggests, as do other contributors, numerous interventions.

At the top of any list of challenges that are also opportunities belongs improving the feedback students receive on the progress they are making — or not — in their professional development. To be of maximum value, feedback and evaluations need to be timely, based on firsthand observations of remediable behavior, and undertaken in a collaborative spirit. But honest, supportive critiques take time; a shortage of this essential element probably explains in part the attendings' shortcomings cited above.

But lack of time is certainly not the only culprit. Useful critiques also require a "safe" environment. Too often students are wary of expressing needs and questions out of the fear of appearing weak or of "rocking the boat" (e.g., "I shouldn't have caused that patient so much pain"). Such questions may become unresolved ethical dilemmas and sources of continuing discomfort rather than sources of learning (Bickel, 1996). Fortunately for those who fly, airline pilots share their questions and errors with each other, understanding this process to be an essential learning device. In his study of surgeons, Bosk (1979) found that the best had the ability to rethink everything that they'd done and imagine how they might have done it differently (Bosk, 1979). Think of the learning and improvements that could occur if all physicians became braver in discussing their mistakes with their colleagues and students.

—————

An overarching theme of this book is the disconnect between what medical educators profess and what students experience. As Hafferty asks here, "If medicine truly harbors [a] 'fundamental specialness' . . . where can we go within the training process to see this essence being nurtured?" Wear (1997) similarly concludes that "we must examine . . . the fit . . . between how we act and what we say is important" (p. 1057). Mission-based management may assist institutions in understanding the true costs of their missions and in making wiser decisions about what to subsidize (Watson & Romrell, 1999; Cohen, 1998). A simpler approach that can be undertaken at the departmental level is faculty workload assessment, to realistically determine expectations and to balance demands against resources (Poehlman, 1999). Such moves toward greater organizational accountability can heighten the recognition that time must be allocated for scholarly and teaching activities and faculty development needs.

But teaching the intricacies of empathic patient care, modeling professional values, and giving effective feedback will never be efficient processes and do not lend themselves to productivity analyses. Leaders must use every means at their disposal to inspire the valuing of these crucial activities, and Reiser, Hafferty, and other contributors suggest many levers.

Evaluation systems certainly ought to reflect far more significantly the importance of professionalism and mentoring. Students can evaluate faculty and faculty can evaluate department chairs on such items as "provides timely feedback," "demonstrates respectful attitudes," and "provides guidance on professional ethics." In this volume Grady-Weliky and colleagues suggest an even bolder formalization of criteria for mentoring in the faculty promotions process: As promotions committees count first authorships in major journals toward full professorships, why not also require a certain number of *last* authorships with mentees as first authors? A less radical step in the right direction would be to require that on each faculty member's annual evaluation, senior faculty list their protégés while trainees and junior faculty name their mentors and role models. Some schools are also facilitating mentor-protégé pairings and offering mentor-of-the-year awards (Bickel, in press).

Actually the fates of students and junior clinical faculty and the future of academic medicine are intimately intertwined. Junior faculty have been hardest hit by imperatives to increase clinical loads. Simultaneously, many are endeavoring to build a research program and to hone skills as scholars and educators — all very time-intensive enterprises. These demands are peaking when most junior faculty also have young children. No wonder many highly committed (and often still in debt) junior faculty are becoming demoralized and leaving academic medicine. Skeff and Mutha (1998) observe that "teachers, even those who are motivated and highly skilled, cannot accomplish these goals [of commitment to the needs of medical students] without institutional support" (p. 2016). If too many students draw too many negative conclusions from the examples of overwhelmed junior faculty, academic medicine will have "eaten its seed corn." What then will become of the "academic" in academic medicine?

As subsidies for medical education evaporate, will drought conditions prevail or will educators rededicate themselves to nurturing students' professional development and social consciences? Actually, even in eras when federal and state "water" and "fertilizer" were more plentiful, medical schools did relatively little to foster the blossoming of a community orientation. Coulehan and Williams chart Andrea's transformation from "eager to get involved . . . and commit[ed] to the well-being of others" to "numb" and believing that "most projects are Band-Aid treatments [that] simply provide an opportunity to feel good about oneself that isn't justified." This loss of eager commitment is especially unfortunate, given that most academic medical centers are near, if not in, an economically deprived area, with no shortage of options for students to acquire "knowledge of and sensitivity to the socioeconomic, emotional and community factors that affect the health and well-being of many patients, especially those . . . in the lower end of the income distribution and who generally have less education, less stable family structures, and fewer social supports" (Ginzberg, 1997, p. 664). Cohen (1999c) similarly singles out medical education's insufficient attention to the needs of the underserved and the erosion of trust between patient and physicians as evidence that medical education and society's expectations are seriously misaligned. Indeed, Frankford and Konrad (1998) argue that "professionalism can survive only if it is . . . responsive to society" (p. 142). They recommend that "traditional individualistic professional autonomy is no longer a viable path; in the face of market imperatives, professionalism can survive only if it is reformulated . . . [to] be more explicitly responsive to society" (p. 144).

A critical element of fitting medical education more precisely to societal needs is preparing physicians to work more effectively as team members. Medicine has tended to attract individuals with a preference for autonomy and control and a tendency to act as "chief." But physicians must increasingly collaborate as equals with nonphysician providers of many types. They must become better at facilitating consensus and at sharing decision making within diverse alliances and within the "new health care team" (Carlson, 1999). And while it has been clear for years that "health care consumers" are more highly informed and expect a more egalitarian relationship with physicians, instead of improving their collaborative skills, many physicians remain stuck in the "control" mode.

The growing heterogeneity of medical students — in terms of gender, ethnicity, age, and previous work experience — may be a positive development here. Even though African Americans, Hispanics, and Native Americans remain woefully underrepresented, the otherwise growing diversity of medical students may facilitate their comfort in working with mixed teams and with diverse populations. This heterogeneity, however, does present extra challenges in terms of the mentoring of students. As Grady-Weliky and colleagues point out, in order to mentor students unlike themselves, our relatively homogeneous faculty need "mentor development programs" including basics in young adult development and support in establishing lasting mentoring alliances.

Women, now 43 percent of medical students, do have a harder time than men garnering the mentoring they need. This undermentoring is particularly unfortunate in view of the promising characteristics they add to the profession. For example, twice as high a proportion of women graduating seniors as men plan to locate in socioeconomically deprived areas, and a higher proportion of women than men follow through on their plans (Bickel & Ruffin, 1995). Crandall and colleagues (1993) likewise found that while the willingness of male students to provide indigent care decreased during medical school, female students' willingness did not decline. In general, studies find that, compared to male physicians, female physicians' encounters with patients include more positive talk, time listening, partnership building, information giving, and emotional support (Elderkin-Thompson & Waitzkin, 1999). Patients of both sexes report that visits to women physicians are more participatory than to those to men (Cooper-

Patrick et al., 1999). These findings are consonant with Lipman-Blumen's observations about women leaders in general:

> Women have lived in *embedded* roles, roles intimately interwoven into the warp and woof of the social context . . . serving as links between other roles, between generations, between institutions, between the public and private domains. . . . Consequently women are no newcomers to the complications generated by interdependence and diversity. (Lipman-Blumen, 1996, pp. 289–90)

Finally, there are encouraging trends in medical education toward problem-based learning and toward the incorporation of women's health into the curriculum. Both require interdisciplinary bridges and teamwork, actually furthering a sense of community within academic medical centers. And adding a focus on women's health also frequently incorporates a more holistic and community-based orientation into the curriculum (Donoghue, 1996).

There is a lot of room for improvement. On AAMC's 1998 Medical School Graduation Questionnaire, high percentages of students rated critical areas as inadequately covered in the curriculum. For instance, 33 percent of men and 41 percent of women seniors thought that time devoted to "public health and community medicine" was inadequate. With regard to the "role of community health and social service agencies," 42 percent and 51 percent, respectively, thought that the time was inadequate; and for "women's health," 27 percent and 37 percent.

A recent compendium of activities to improve the social responsiveness of medical schools around the world (Gary et al., 1999) reveals an encouraging and expanding breadth of activity. Our book provides but a few examples of community-campus partnerships. Actually, the number of ongoing community-based outreach services fostered by academic medical centers resists cataloging. Pawlson's (1998) overview names an extensive range, from activities closely related to clinical services (e.g., mobile vans for mammography, health fairs, and health advocacy programs, such as firearm safety) to community health-needs assessment and demonstration programs to school-based health education to targeted services for special occupations (e.g., prisoners, the homeless, migrants, pregnant women).

Service-learning programs might be considered a subset of such partnerships, that is, "structured learning experience that combines community service with explicit learning objectives, preparation and reflection" (Seifer, 1998). Service learning is developed, implemented, and evaluated in collaboration with the community and responds to community-identified concerns. At least seventeen health professions schools (including Rush, as described by Eckenfels here) have integrated service learning into the curriculum, conduct faculty development training in service learning, and directly involve community members in curriculum implementation. Less-comprehensive but innovative programs are regularly reported in *Academic Medicine* and elsewhere, such as the University of West Virginia School of Medicine's "clinical learning groups" focusing on the patient, the physician, and the community (Antonelli & Cutlip, 1999) and the University of Tennessee College of Medicine's required longitudinal community clinical program (Thompson et al., 1999).

One important feature of service-learning programs is that they build in critical reflection, to facilitate students' connection between the service experience and their learning. Reflective practice is encouraged through discussions led by "community mentors" and through journal keeping and engaging in dialogues. Novack and colleagues (1999) have stressed that "reflection-in-action" is fundamental to professional growth and offer a variety of examples of how medical educators can better foster self-awareness in their students in all settings.

—————

That medical students are learning when we least expect it is both our greatest challenge and greatest opportunity. Naturally, we tend to focus on the defoliating aspects of the current climate. But witness how many of the activities discussed in this book are student generated, and how excited our authors are to share their experiences as assistant gardeners.

Excitement may be too much to ask of our generally overextended junior clinical faculty, however. What about leaning more heavily on our senior faculty? While they too have full plates, most earn enviable salaries and have greater security and access to resources and more time than their younger colleagues. Faculty stuck in gloom and doom and in "doctor knows best" may be irredeemable. But most schools have untapped wealth in their faculty — individuals ready to give of their strengths to nourish the "seeds" in their midst. Medical schools can better stimulate and facilitate senior faculty members' participation in students' professional development, in institutional improvements, and in public service and community partnerships. Some emeritus professors have energy and commitment to contribute as well, such as the two emeritus professors at Stanford who are co-leading an innovative faculty-mentoring program.

Finally, deans, department heads, and other senior administrators — the norm setters and reward apportioners — carry the heaviest responsibilities, not only for the bottom line but also for professionalism and community service. As leadership challenges increase, how will academic medicine recruit individuals who will fill this tall bill? An executive search process that focuses above all on a candidate's scientific and money-generating expertise is dangerously narrow. Medical centers need to work to assure that they are attracting leaders who will give "conspicuous and credible priority" not only to fiscal management but also to compassion and respect (Burack et al., 1999, p. 54). A medical school may get the leaders it deserves, but what about the patients its graduates serve?

Members of the medical profession must become more explicitly responsive to societal needs or lose their struggle for identity as patient advocates. Sulmasy (1999) reminds us that this identity struggle is contributing to "how much physicians are suffering today" (p. 1004). As confounding as the current cutbacks, profiteering, and mergers are, Sulmasy also reminds us that the "spiritual meaning of medicine will outlast all mergers" (p. 1004). One anodyne is a reconnection with the spiritual, for instance, more dialogue among physicians who ask the following questions: "What is the meaning of medicine? What are good healing relationships about? Can we move beyond kvetching about the pressures we now face? Can we see our work as service?" (p. 1004). Such questions lie at the core of professionalism and reveal the synergy between social conscience and the engagement of the spirit.

These perilous times require that each — from student to dean — be ever developing as professionals, as communicators, as leaders. Communities *expect* leadership from physicians. And no wonder. No group is better equipped to champion improvements in the health care system. While competition and restrictions may be mounting, physicians are the ones with the greatest access to knowledge of the human body, to medical technology and resources, and to the respect of those they serve. If courageous and compassionate, each physician has enormous potential for positive impact. This book offers a wealth of ideas on better realizing these potentials. Opportunities do abound.

REFERENCES

American Board of Internal Medicine. (1992). *Guide to awareness and evaluation of humanistic qualities in the internist*. Philadelphia, PA: American Board of Internal Medicine.

American Board of Internal Medicine. (1995). *Project professionalism*. Philadelphia, PA: American Board of Internal Medicine.

American Board of Internal Medicine. (1999). *Project Professionalism*. Philadelphia, PA: American Board of Internal Medicine.

American Medical Association. (1997). *AMA policy compendium*. Chicago, IL: American Medical Association.

American Medical Association, Council on Ethical and Judicial Affairs. (1995). Ethical issues in managed care. *Journal of the American Medical Association, 273*, 330–335.

American Medical Association, Council on Ethical and Judicial Affairs. (1996). *Code of medical ethics: Current opinions with annotations*. Chicago, IL: American Medical Association.

Anders, G., & McGinley, L. (1997, April 1). A new brand of crime now stirs the Feds: Health-care fraud: Enforcement budgets rise as agencies train sights on big, complex cases: "Killed on the hospice story." *Wall Street Journal*, pp. A1, A8.

Anderson, R. A., & Obenshian, S. S. (1994). Cheating by students: Findings, reflections, and remedies. *Academic Medicine, 69*, 323–331.

Andre, J. (1991). Beyond moral reasoning: A wider view of the professional ethics course. *Teaching Philosophy, 14(4)*, 359–373.

Andre, J. (1992). Learning to see: Moral growth during medical school. *Journal of Medical Ethics, 18*, 148–152.

Antonelli, M. A. S., & Cutlip, A. D. (1999). A first-year course focused on the patient, the physician, and the community. *Academic Medicine, 74*, 599–600.

Arnold, E. L., Blank, L., Race, K. H., & Cipparrone, N. (1998). Can professionalism be measured? The development of a scale for use in the medical environment. *Academic Medicine, 73*, 1119–1121.

Aron, R. (1967). *Main currents in sociological thought*. New York, NY: Basic Books.

Association of American Medical Colleges. (1984). *Physicians for the twenty-first century: The GPEP report*. Washington, DC: Association of American Medical Colleges.

Association of American Medical Colleges. (1998). *Learning objectives for medical student education: Guidelines for medical schools. Medical school objectives project* (Report 1). Washington, DC: Association of American Medical Colleges.

Bacik, J. (1996). *Spirituality in transition*. Kansas City, MO: Sheed & Ward.

Baker, R. (1993). Deciphering Percival's code. In R. Baker, D. Porter, & R. Porter (Eds.), *The codification of medical morality* (pp. 179–211). Netherlands: Kluwer Academic Publishers.

Baldwin, D. C., Daugherty, S. R., & Rowley, B. D. (1998). Unethical and unprofessional conduct observed by residents during their first year of training. *Academic Medicine, 73*, 1195–1200.

Barber, B. (1963). Some problems in the sociology of the professions. *Daedalus, 92*, 669–688.

Barer, M. L., & Stoddart, G. L. (1992). Toward integrated medical resource policies for Canada: Undergraduate medical training. *Canadian Medical Association Journal, 147*, 305–312.

Barzun, J. (1978). The professions under siege. *Harpers, 236*, 231–236, 268.

Bayles, M. D. (1989). *Medical ethics*. Belmont, CA: Wadsworth.

Becker, H., Geer, B., Hughes, E. C., & Strauss, A. L. (1961). *Boys in white: Student culture in medical school*. Chicago, IL: University of Chicago Press.

Benjamin, M. (1990). *Splitting the difference: Compromise and integrity in ethics and politics*. Lawrence, KS: University Press of Kansas.

Berger, P. L. (1963). *Invitation to sociology: A humanistic perspective*. New York, NY: Doubleday Anchor Books.

Berger, P. L., & Luckman, T. (1966). *The social construction of reality*. New York, NY: Doubleday.

Berkman, L. (1984). Assessing the physical health effects of social networks and social support. *Annual Review of Public Health, 5*, 413–432.

Bickel, J. (1987). Human values teaching programs in the clinical education of medical students. *Journal of Medical Education, 62*, 369–378.

Bickel, J. (1996). Proceedings of the AAMC conference on students' and residents' ethical and professional development. *Academic Medicine, 71(6)*, 622–642.

Bickel, J. (2000). *Women in medicine: Getting in, surviving, and advancing*. Thousand Oaks, CA: Sage Publications.

Bickel, J., & Ruffin, A. (1995). Gender-associated differences in matriculating and graduating medical students. *Academic Medicine, 70*, 552–559.

Bloom, S. (1963). The process of becoming a physician. *Annals of the American Academy of Political and Social Sciences, 346*, 77–87.

Bloom, S. W. (1963). The doctor and his patient: A sociological interpretation. New York: Russell Sage Foundation.

Bloom, S. W. (1989). The medical school as a social organization: the sources of resistance to change. *Medical Education, 23*, 228–241.

Bloomquist, J. (1997). Holy time, holy timing. *Weavings: A Journal of the Christian Spiritual Life, 6(1)*, 7–13.

Bosk, C. L. (1979). *Forgive and remember: Managing medical failure*. Chicago, IL: University of Chicago Press.

Bosk, C. L. (1992). *All God's mistakes: Genetic counseling in a pediatric hospital*. Chicago, IL: University of Chicago Press.

Bradley, F. H. (1988). *Ethical studies*. Oxford, UK: Clarendon Press.

Brennan, T. A., Leape, L. L., Laird, N. M., Hebert, L., Localio, A. R., Lawthers, A. G., Newhouse, J. P., Weiler, P. C., & Hiatt, H. H. (1991). Incidence of adverse events and negligence in hospitalized patients — results of the Harvard medical practice study 1. *New England Journal of Medicine, 324*, 370–376.

Bridging the Gaps: Philadelphia Community Health Internship Program. (1996). *1996 health action report*. (Available from BTG Program Office, Room 911 Blockley Hall, 423 Guardian Drive, Philadelphia, PA 19104).

Bridging the Gaps: Philadelphia Community Health Internship Program. (1997). *1997 health action report*. (Available from BTG Program Office, Room 911 Blockley Hall, 423 Guardian Drive, Philadelphia, PA 19104).

Bridging the Gaps Network. (1998). *1998 program evaluation*. (Available from Bridging the Gaps Program Office, Room 911 Blockley Hall, 423 Guardian Drive, Philadelphia, PA 19104).

Brody, H. (1992). *The healer's power*. New Haven, CT: Yale University Press.

Brody, H., Squier, H. A., & Foglio, J. P. (1995). Commentary: Moral growth in medical students. *Theoretical Medicine, 16*, 281–289.

Burack, J. H., Irby, D. M., Carline, J. D., Root, R. K., and Larson, E. B. (1999). Teaching compassion and respect: Attending physicians' responses to problematic behaviors. *Journal of General Internal Medicine, 14*, 49–55.

Buxbaum, R. (1997). *Aging well: A theological perspective*. Philadelphia, PA: Board of Pensions, Presbyterian Church USA.

Camanisch, P. F. (1988). On being a professional, morally speaking. In A. Flores (Ed.), *Professional ideals* (pp. 14–37). Belmont, CA: Wadsworth.

Carlson, B. (1999). The new health care team. *Physician Executive, 25*, 67–75.

Carr, J. E. (1994). Basic behavioral science in medical education: The need for reform. *Annals of Behavioral Science and Medical Education, 1(1)*, 5–13.

Cassell, E. J. (1991). *The nature of suffering and the goals of medicine*. New York, NY: Oxford University Press.

Cato 6. (1982). Dirtball. *Journal of the American Medical Association, 247*, 3059–3060.

Christakis, D. A. (1995). The similarity and frequency of proposals to reform U.S. medical education: Constant concerns. *Journal of the American Medical Association, 274*, 706–711.

Christakis, D. A. (1996). Characteristics of the informal curriculum and trainees' ethical choices. In J. Bickel (Ed.), Proceedings of the AAMC conference on students' and residents' ethical and professional development (pp. 631–633). *Academic Medicine, 71*, 621–642.

Christakis, D. A., & Feudtner, C. (1993). Ethics in a short white coat: A report on the ethical dilemmas that medical students confront. *Academic Medicine, 68*, 249–254.

Christakis, D. A., & Feudtner, C. (1997). Temporary matters: The ethical consequences of transient social relationships in medical training. *Journal of the American Medical Association, 278*, 739–743.

Clancy, C. M., & Brody, H. (1995). Managed care: Jekyll or Hyde? *Journal of the American Medical Association, 273(4)*, 338–339.

Claxton, G. (1997). *Hare brain tortoise mind*. Hopewell, NJ: Ecco Press.

Cohen, J. J. (1998). Mission-based management: Lessons from the real world. *Academic Medicine, 73*, 982.

Cohen, J. J. (1998a). Leadership for medicine's promising future. *Academic Medicine, 73*, 132–137.

Cohen, J. J. (1998b). From the president: People want their doctors back. *Academic Medicine, 73*, 772.

Cohen, J. J. (1998c, October 30–November 5). Honoring the "E" in GME. An address given at the 109th Association of American Medical Colleges annual meeting, New Orleans, Louisiana.

Cohen, J. J. (1999a). Honoring the "E" in GME. *Academic Medicine, 74*, 108–112.

Cohen, J. J. (1999b). Lining up with students against abuse. *Academic Medicine, 74*, 45.

Cohen, J. J. (1999c). Missions of a medical school: A North American perspective. *Academic Medicine, 74*, S27–S30.

Coles, R. (1993). *The call of service: A witness to idealism*. New York, NY: Houghton Mifflin.

Coles, R. (1998). The moral education of medical students. *Academic Medicine, 73*, 55–57.

Collins, R. (1979). *The credential society*. New York, NY: Academic Press.

Conrad, P. (1988). Learning to doctor: Reflections on recent accounts of the medical school years. *Journal of Health and Social Behavior, 29*, 323–332.

Coombs, R. H., Chopra, S., Schenk, D., & Yutan, E. (1993). Medical slang and its functions. *Social Science and Medicine, 36*, 987–998.

Cooper-Patrick, L., Gallo, J., Gonzales, J., Vu, H. T., Pows, N., & Ford, D. E. (1999). Race, gender and partnership in the patient-physician relationship. *Journal of the American Medical Association, 282*, 583–589.

Coulehan, J. L. (1996). Tenderness and steadiness: Emotions in medical practice. *Literature and Medicine, 14*, 222–236.

Coulehan, J. L. (1997). Being a physician. In M. B. Mengel & W. L. Holleman (Eds.), *Fundamentals of clinical practice: A textbook on the patient, doctor, and society* (pp. 73–101). New York: Plenum Publishing Company.

Coulehan, J. L., Williams, P. C., Landis, D., & Naser, C. (1995). The first patient: Reflections and stories about the anatomy cadaver. *Teaching and Learning in Medicine, 7*, 61–66.

Coulehan, J. L., Williams, P. C., & Naser, C. (1995). The virtual group: Electronic mail in teaching medical humanities. *Academic Medicine, 70*, 158–160.

Covey, S. R. (1989). *Seven habits of highly effective people: Restoring the character ethic*. New York: Fireside.

Crandall, S., Volk, R., Loemker, V. (1993). Medical students' attitudes toward providing care for the underserved. *Journal of the American Medical Association, 269*, 2519–2523.

Crawshaw, R., Rogers, D. E., Pellegrino, E. D., Bulger, R. J., Lundberg, G. D., Bristow, L. R., Cassel, C. K., & Barondess, J. A. (1995). Patient-physician covenant. *Journal of the American Medical Association, 273*, 1553.

Crigger, B. J. (1998). What could have saved John Worthy? *Hastings Center Report, 28(4)*, S1–S18.

Cruess, R. L., & Cruess, S. (1997). Teaching medicine as a profession in the service of healing. *Academic Medicine, 72*, 941–952.

Curry, R., & Makoul, G. (1998). The evolution of courses in professional skills and perspectives for medical students. *Academic Medicine, 73*, 10–13.

Cwiklik, R. (1998, February 6). A different course: For many people, college will no longer be a specific place, or a specific time. *Wall Street Journal*, pp. R31, R33.

Davis, R. (1998, October 28). Report urges studying medical errors. *USA Today*, p. 4A.

Doctor X. (1965). *Intern*. New York, NY: Harper and Row.

Donoghue, G. (Ed.) (1996). *Women's health in the curriculum: A resource for faculty*. Philadelphia, PA: National Academy of Women's Health Medical Education (Medical College of Pennsylvania/Hahnemann University).

Drane, J. F. (1988). *Becoming a good doctor: The place of virtue and character in medical ethics*. Kansas City, MO: Sheed & Ward.

Dubovsky, S. L. (1987). Coping with entitlement in medical education. *New England Journal of Medicine, 315*, 1672–1674.

Duncan, D. E. (1996). *Residents: The perils and promises of educating young doctors*. New York, NY: Scribner.

Dwyer, J. (1994). Primum non tacere: An ethics of speaking up. *Hastings Center Report, 24(1)*, 13–18.

References

Eckenfels, E. J. (1993). Student-faculty collaboration to enhance community health. In W. D. Skelton & M. Osterweis (Eds.), *Promoting community health — the role of the academic health center* (pp. 199–210). Washington, DC: Association of Academic Health Centers.

Eckenfels, E. J. (1997). Contemporary medical students' quest for self-fulfillment through community service. *Academic Medicine, 72*, 1043–1050.

Eckenfels, E. J., Baier, C., Turner-Roan, K., & Sanchez, A. M. (1994). *Enhancing the learning and development of medical students through community service. Effective learning, effective teaching, effective service: Three voices from the field on improving education through community-service learning.* Washington, DC: Your Service America's Working Group on National and Community Service Policy.

Educating Future Physicians for Ontario. (1993). Part 1 summary: What people of Ontario need and expect from physicians. Hamilton, Ont.: EFPO Co-ordinating Centre.

Eisenberg, L. (1979). A friend, not an apple, will keep the doctor away. *Journal of the American Medical Association, 66*, 551–553.

Eisler, P., & Pearson, B. (1999, February 23). Feds triple health fraud cases: Crackdown hits Medicare billing abuses. *USA Today*, pp. 1A, 5B.

Elderkin-Thompson, V., & Waitzkin, H. (1999). Differences in clinical communication by gender. *Journal of General Internal Medicine, 14*, 112–121.

Emanuel, L. (1997). Bringing market medicine to professional accountability. *Journal of the American Medical Association, 277*, 1004–1005.

Emmett, R. I. (1995). A descriptive analysis of medical school application forms. *Academic Medicine, 68*, 564–569.

Eng, E., Salmon, M., & Mullan, F. (1992). Community empowerment: The critical base for primary health care. *Family Community Health, 15*, 1–12.

Engel, G. L. (1977). The need for a new medical model: A challenge for biomedicine. *Science, 196*, 129–136.

Erde, E. L. (1997). The inadequacy of role models for educating medical students in ethics with some reflections on virtue theory. *Theoretical Medicine, 18*, 31–45.

Fetzer Institute. (1998). *The institute report.* Kalamazoo, MI: Fetzer Institute.

Feudtner, C., & Christakis, D. A. (1994). Making the rounds: The ethical development of medical students in the context of clinical rotations. *Hastings Center Report, 24(1)*, 6–12.

Feudtner, C., Christakis, D. A., & Christakis, N. A. (1994). Do clinical clerks suffer ethical erosion? Students' perceptions of their clinical environment and personal development. *Academic Medicine, 69*, 670–679.

Fields, S. A., Toffler, W., Elliot, D., & Chappelle, K. (1998). Principles of clinical medicine: Oregon Health Sciences University School of Medicine. *Academic Medicine, 73*, 25–31.

Flach, D. H., Smith, M. F., Smith, W. G., & Glasser, M. L. (1982). Faculty mentors for medical students. *Journal of Medical Education, 57*, 514–520.

Flores, A. (1988). *Professional ideals.* Belmont, CA: Wadsworth.

Forrow, L., & Wolf, M. L. (1998). Ideals in action: The U.S. Schweitzer Fellows Programs. *Academic Medicine, 73*, 658–661.

Foster, G. S. (1998). Truth and consequences. *Academic Medicine, 73*, 1226–1227.

Fox, R. (1988). *Essays in medical sociology: Journeys into the field.* New Brunswick, NJ: Transaction Press.

Frankford, D. M., & Konrad, T. R. (1998). Responsive medical professionalism: Integrating education, practice, and community in a market-driven era. *Academic Medicine, 73*, 138–145.

Frankl, V. (1959). *From death camp to existentialism: A psychiatrist's path to new therapy*. Boston, MA: Beacon Press.

Freidson, E. (1994). *Professionalism reborn: Theory, prophecy, and policy*. Chicago, IL: University of Chicago Press.

Fried, L. P., Francomano, C. A., MacDonald, S. M., Wagner, E. M., Stokes, E. J., Carbone, K. M., Bias, W. B., Newman, M. M., & Stobo, J. D. (1996). Career development for women in academic medicine: Multiple interventions in a department of medicine. *Journal of the American Medical Association, 276(11)*, 898–905.

Liaison Committee on Medical Education. (1998). Functions and structure of a medical school. Washington, DC: Association of American Medical Colleges.

Gary, N., Boelen, C., Gastel, B., & Ayers, W. (Eds.) (1999). Improving the social responsiveness of medical schools. Proceedings of the 1998 Educational Commission for Foreign Medical Graduates/World Health Organization Invitational Conference. *Academic Medicine, 74*, Sviii–S94.

Ginzberg, E. (1997). Medical education and the needs of the public. *Academic Medicine, 72*, 663–665.

Glick, S. (1981). Humanistic medicine in a modern age. *New England Journal of Medicine, 304(17)*, 1036–1038.

Goe, L. C., Merrera, A. M., & Mower, W. R. (1998). Misrepresentation of research citations among medical school faculty applicants. *Academic Medicine, 73*, 1183–1186.

Arnold P. Gold Foundation (1997, November). Challenging the barriers to sustaining humanism in medicine (2d Barriers symposium). Lake Forest, IL. Unpublished proceedings.

Arnold P. Gold Foundation (1998, June). Challenging the barriers to sustaining humanism in medicine (3rd Barriers symposium). Alexandria, VA. Unpublished proceedings.

Good, B. J. (1994). *Medicine, rationality, and experience: An anthropological perspective*. New York, NY: Cambridge University Press.

Good, M.-J. D. V., & Good, B. J. (1989). Disabling practitioners: Hazards of learning to be a doctor in American medical education. *Journal of Orthopsychiatry, 59*, 303–309.

Goode, W. J. (1969). *The theoretical limits of professionalization*. New York, NY: Free Press.

Gordon, M. J. (1997). Cutting the gordian knot: A two-part approach to the evaluation and professional development of residents. *Academic Medicine, 72*, 876–880.

Goulet, D. (1971). An ethical model for the study of values. *Harvard Educational Review, 41*, 205–227.

Gray, B. H. (1997). Trust and trustworthy care in the managed care era. *Health Affairs, 16*, 34–49.

Group Health Association of America. (1994). *Primary care physicians: Recommendations to reform medical education. Competencies needed to practice in HMOs*. Washington, DC: Group Health Association of America.

Guglielmo, W. J. (1998). Are D.O.'s losing their unique identity? *Medical Economics, 75(8)*, 200–214.

Gula, R. (1996). *Ethics in pastoral ministry*. New York, NY: Paulist Press.

Gupta, A. R., Duffy, T. P., & Johnston, M. A. (1997). Incorporating multiculturalism into a doctor-patient course. *Academic Medicine, 72*, 428.

Haas, J., & Shaffir, W. (1982a). Taking the role of doctor: A dramaturgical analysis of professionalization. *Symbolic Interaction, 5*, 187–203.

Haas, J., & Shaffir, W. (1982b). Ritual evaluation of competence: The hidden curriculum of professionalization in an innovative medical school program. *Work and Occupations, 9*, 131–154.

Hafferty, F. W. (1991, August 23–27). Trust, ideology, and professional power. Presentation to the American Sociological Association, Eighty-sixth annual meeting, Cincinnati, OH.

Hafferty, F. W. (1998). Beyond curriculum reform: Confronting medicine's hidden curriculum. *Academic Medicine, 73*, 403–407.

Hafferty, F. W. (1999). Medical education. In C. Bird, P. Conrad, & A. Fremont (Eds.), *Handbook of Medical Sociology* (5th ed.). New York, NY: Prentice Hall.

Hafferty, F. W., & Franks, R. (1994). The hidden curriculum, ethics teaching, and the structure of medical education. *Academic Medicine, 69*, 861–871.

Hafferty, F. W., & Light, D. W. (1995). Professional dynamics and the changing nature of medical work. *Journal of Health and Social Behavior* (special ed.), 132–153.

Hafferty, F. W., & McKinlay, J. B. (1993a). *The changing medical profession: An international perspective*. New York, NY: Oxford University Press.

Hafferty, F. W., & McKinlay, J. B. (1993b). Conclusion: Cross-cultural perspectives on the dynamics of medicine as a profession. In F. W. Hafferty & J. B. McKinlay (Eds.), *The changing medical profession: An international perspective* (pp. 210–226). New York, NY: Oxford University Press.

Hahn, R. A., Eaker, E., Barker, N. D., Teutsch, S. M., Sosniak, W., & Krieger, N. (1995). Poverty and death in the United States — 1973 and 1991. *Epidemiology, 6*, 490–497.

Hampson, R. (1995, March 18). Hospital horror stories: Trend or the exception? *Duluth News-Tribune*, pp. 1A, 6A.

Haug, M. R. (1988). A re-examination of the hypothesis of physician deprofessionalization. *Milbank Quarterly, 66*, 48–56.

Heagerty, B. V. (n.d.). Medical education and the struggle for reform: The College of Human Medicine. Unpublished manuscript, Michigan State University.

Hensel, W. A., & Dickey, N. W. (1998). Teaching professionalism: Passing the torch. *Academic Medicine, 73*, 865–870.

Herzberg, G. L. (1998). Student perceptions of the value of medical ethics education. Unpublished doctoral dissertation, University of Michigan.

Hiatt, J. F. (1986). Spirituality, medicine and healing. *Southern Medical Journal, 79(6)*, 736–743.

Hilfiker, D. (1987). *Healing the wounds*. New York, NY: Viking Penguin.

Hilts, P. J. (1991, December 4). Science and the stain of scandal. *New York Times*, p. B1.

Hippocrates (1923a). The oath. In W. H. S. Jones (Ed.), *Hippocrates: Vol. 1* (pp. 299–301). Cambridge, MA: Harvard University Press.

Hippocrates. (1923b). The physician. In W. H. S. Jones (Ed.), *Hippocrates: Vol. 2* (pp. 311–313). Cambridge, MA: Harvard University Press.

Hoffmann, S. (1990). *Under the ether dome: A physician's apprenticeship*. New York, NY: Citadel Press.

Holleman, W. L., Holleman, M. C., & Moy, J. G. (1997). Are ethics and managed care strange bedfellows or a marriage made in heaven? *Lancet, 349*, 350–351.

Hughes, R. G., Barker, D. C., & Reynolds, R. C. (1994). Are we mortgaging the medical profession? *New England Journal of Medicine, 326*, 274–275.

Hundert, E. M. (1996). Characteristics of the informal curriculum and trainees' ethical choices. *Academic Medicine, 71*, 624–633.

Hundert, E. M. (1997, October 18–21). *The role of the hidden curriculum in the professional development of medical students.* Paper presented at the Association for Behavioral Sciences and Medical Education, Twenty-seventh annual meeting, Brewster, MA.

Hundert, E. M. (1998, October 30–November 5). *The powerful creditless curriculum.* A plenary address given at the 109th Association of American Medical Colleges annual meeting, New Orleans, LA.

Hundert, E. M., Douglas-Steele, D., & Bickel, J. (1996). Context in medical education: The informal ethics curriculum. *Medical Education, 30*, 353–364.

Hunt, A. (1991). *Medical education, accreditation and the nation's health: Reflections of an atypical dean.* New York, NY: McGraw Hill.

Hunt, A. D., & Brody, H. (1983). Medical humanities at Michigan State University. *Mobius, 2(3)*, 81–88.

Hunt, A. D., & Weeks, L. E. (Eds.). (1979). *Medical education since 1960: Marching to a different drummer.* East Lansing, MI: Michigan State University Foundation.

Hunter, K. M., Charon, R., & Coulehan, J. L. (1995). The study of literature in medical education. *Academic Medicine, 70*, 787–794.

Igartua, K. (1997). Fostering faculty mentorship of junior medical students. *Academic Medicine, 72(1)*, 3.

Illich, I. (1976). *Medical nemesis: The expropriation of our health.* New York, NY: Pantheon.

Inui, T. S. (1992). The social contract and the medical school's responsibilities. In K. L. White & J. E. Connelly (Eds.), *The medical school's mission and the population's health* (pp. 23–59). New York, NY: Springer Verlag.

Jameton, A. (1993). Dilemmas of moral distress: Moral responsibility and nursing practice. *Clinical Issues in Perinatal and Women's Health Nursing, 4(4)*, 542–551.

Johnston, M. A. (1992). A model program to address insensitive behaviors toward medical students. *Academic Medicine, 67*, 236–237.

Jonas, S. (1978). *Medical mystery: The training of doctors in the United States.* New York, NY: W. W. Norton & Company.

Kark, S. (1981). *The practice of community-oriented primary health care.* New York, NY: Appleton-Century-Crofts.

Kassebaum, D. G., & Cutler, E. R. (1998). On the culture of student abuse in medical schools. *Academic Medicine, 73*, 1149–1158.

Kassebaum, D. G., Cutler, E. R., & Eaglen, R. H. (1997). The influence of accreditation on educational change in U.S. medical schools. *Academic Medicine, 72*, 1127–1133.

Kassebaum, D. G., Eaglen, R. H., & Cutler, E. R. (1997). The objectives of medical education: Reflections in the accreditation looking glass. *Academic Medicine, 72*, 647–656.

Kassirer, J. P. (1998). Managing care: Should we adopt a new ethic? *New England Journal of Medicine, 339*, 397–398.

Kaufman, A., Galbraith, P., Alfero, C., Urbina, C., Derksen, D., Wiese, W., Contreras, R., & Kalishman, N. (1996). Fostering the health of communities: A unifying mission for the University of New Mexico Health Sciences Center. *Academic Medicine, 71*, 432–440.

Kaufman, J. S., Cooper, R. S., & McGee, D. L. (1997). Socioeconomic status and health in blacks and whites: The problem of residual confounding and the resiliency of race. *Epidemiology, 8*, 621–628.

Klass, P. (1987). *A not entirely benign procedure: Four years as a medical student.* New York, NY: Putnam.

Knight, J. A. (1995). Moral growth in medical students. *Theoretical Medicine, 16*, 265–280.

Kohlberg, L. (1984). *The psychology of moral development: The nature and validity of moral stages.* San Francisco, CA: Harper & Row.

Konner, M. (1987). *Becoming a doctor: A journey of initiation in medical school.* New York, NY: Penguin.

Kretzman, J., & McKnight, J. (1993). *Building communities from the inside out: A path toward finding and mobilizing a community's assets.* Evanston, IL: Institute for Policy Research, Northwestern University. (Distributed by ACTA Publications, Chicago.)

Krieger, N., & Sidney, S. (1996). Racial discrimination and blood pressure: The CARDIA study of young black and white adults. *American Journal of Public Health, 86*, 1370–1378.

Krimerman, L., & Lindenfeld, F. (1992). *When workers decide: Workplace democracy takes root in North America.* Philadelphia, PA: New Society Publishers.

Kultgen, J. (1988). *Ethics and professionalism.* Philadelphia, PA: University of Pennsylvania Press.

Langley, M. (1997, May 2). M.D. VS. M.B.A.: Columbia tells doctors at a hospital to end their outside practices: A showdown nears as physician in Fort Worth refuses administrator's demands: The power shift in medicine. *Wall Street Journal*, pp. A1, A6.

Langreth, R. (1998, August 13). Drug marketing drives many clinical trials. *Wall Street Journal,* p. A10.

Larson, M. S. (1977). *The rise of professionalism: A sociological analysis.* Berkeley, CA: University of California Press.

Lawrance, L., & McLeroy, K. R. (1986). Self-efficacy and health education. *Journal of School Health, 56*, 317–321.

Leake, C. D. (1927). *Percival's medical ethics.* New York, NY: Williams and Wilkins.

Leape, L. L. (1994). Error in medicine. *Journal of the American Medical Association, 272(23),* 1851–1857.

LeBourdais, E. (1994). Physicians cannot be educated in isolation from public concerns, ACMC conference told. *Canadian Medical Association Journal, 151*, 83–85.

Leiderman, D. B., & Grisso, J.-A. (1985). The gomer phenomenon. *Journal of Health and Social Behavior, 26*, 222–232.

Lifton, R. J. (1986). *The Nazi doctors: Medical killing and the psychology of genocide.* New York, NY: Basic Books.

Light, D. W. (1980). *Becoming psychiatrists.* New York, NY: W. W. Norton & Company.

Light, D. W. (1993). *Countervailing power: The changing character of the medical profession in the United States.* New York, NY: Oxford University Press.

Lipman-Blumen, J. (1996). *The connective edge: Leading in an interdependent world.* San Francisco, CA: Jossey Bass.

Luban, D. (1988). *Lawyers and justice: An ethical study.* Princeton, NJ: Princeton University Press.

Ludmerer, K. M. (1985). *Learning to heal: The development of American medical education.* New York, NY: Basic Books.

Lundberg, G. (1990). Countdown to millennium — balancing the professionalism and business of medicine. Medicine's rocking horse. *Journal of the American Medical Association, 263,* 86–87.

Lundberg, G. (1991). Promoting professionalism through self-appraisal in this critical decade. *Journal of the American Medical Association, 265,* 2859.

MacIntyre, A. (1981). *After virtue.* Notre Dame, IN: Notre Dame University Press.

Maheux, B., & Beland, F. (1986). Students' perceptions of values emphasized in three medical schools. *Journal of Medical Education, 61(4),* 308–316.

Makoul, G., & Curry, R. (1998). Patient, physician and society: Northwestern University Medical School. *Academic Medicine, 73,* 140–142.

Makoul, G., Curry, R. H., & Novack, D. H. (1998). The future of medical school courses in professional skills and perspectives. *Academic Medicine, 73,* 48–51.

Manson, A. (1994). The fate of idealism in modern medicine. *Journal of Medical Humanities, 15,* 153–162.

Marion, R. (1989). *The intern blues.* New York, NY: Fawcett Crest Book.

Marion, R. (1991). *Learning to play God.* New York, NY: Fawcett Crest Book.

Marion, R. (1998). *Rotations: The twelve months of intern life.* New York, NY: HarperCollins.

Marston, R. Q., & Jones, R. M. (Eds.). (1992). *Medical education in transition/Commission on medical education: The sciences of medical practice.* Princeton, NJ: Robert Wood Johnson Foundation.

Maudsley, R. F. (1999). Content in context: Medical education and society's needs. *Academic Medicine, 74(2),* 143–145.

May, W. F. (1975). Code, covenant, contract, or philanthropy. *Hastings Center Report, 5,* 29–38.

McArthur, J. H., & Moore, F. D. (1997). The two cultures and the health care revolution. *Journal of the American Medical Association, 277,* 985–989.

McCrorie, P., Lefford, F., & Perrin, F. (1993). Medical undergraduate community-based teaching: A survey for ASME on current and proposed teaching in the community and in general practice in UK universities. ASME Occasional Publication No. 3. Dundee, UK: Association for the Study of Medical Education.

McCurdy, L., Goode, L. D., Inui, T. S., Daugherty, R. M., Jr., Wilson, D. E., Wallace, A. G., Weinstein, B. M., & Copelande, E. M., III. (1997). Fulfilling the social contract between medical schools and the public. *Academic Medicine, 72,* 1063–1070.

McEntyre, M. C. (1997). Getting from how to why: A pause for reflection on professional life. *Academic Medicine, 72,* 1051–1055.

McKinlay, J. B., & Arches, J. (1985). Toward the proletarianization of physicians. *International Journal of Health Services, 15,* 161–195.

McKnight, J. (1997). Two tools for well-being: Health systems and communities. In M. Minkler (Ed.), *Community organizing and community building for health* (pp. 20–29). New Brunswick, NJ: Rutgers University Press.

Mechanic, D. (1985). Physicians and patients in transition. *Hastings Center Report, 15,* 9–12.

Mechanic, D., & Schlesinger, M. (1996). The impact of managed care on patients' trust in medical care and their physicians. *Journal of the American Medical Association, 275,* 1693–1697.

The Medical School Objectives Writing Group. (1999). Learning objectives for medical student education: Guidelines for medical schools. Report 1 of the Medical School Objectives Project. *Academic Medicine, 74,* 13–18.

Merton, R. K., Reader, L. G., & Kendall, P. L. (1957). *The student-physician: Introductory studies in the sociology of medical education.* Cambridge, MA: Harvard University Press.

Merton, T. (1966). *Conjectures of a guilty bystander.* New York, NY: Doubleday.

Meyer, G. S., Potter, A., & Gary, N. (1997). A national survey to define a new core curriculum to prepare physicians for managed care practice. *Academic Medicine, 72,* 669–676.

Michels, R. (1996). Afterword. In E. Ginzberg (Ed.), *Urban medical centers: Balancing academic and patient care functions* (pp. 93–94). Boulder, CO: Westview Press.

Miles, S. H., & Koepp, R. (1995). Comments on the AMA report "Ethical issues in managed care." *Journal of Clinical Ethics, 6,* 306–311.

Miller, F. G., & Brody, H. (1995). Professional integrity and physician-assisted suicide. *Hastings Center Report, 25(3),* 8–17.

Mizrahi, T. (1986). *Getting rid of patients: Contradictions in the socialization of physicians.* New Brunswick, NJ: Rutgers University Press.

Moline, J. N. (1986). Professionals and professions: A philosophical examination of an idea. *Social Science and Medicine, 22,* 501–508.

Montgomery, L. E., Kiely, J. L., & Pappas, G. (1996). The effects of poverty, race, and family structure on U.S. children's health: Data from the NHIS, 1978 through 1980 and 1989 through 1991. *American Journal of Public Health, 86,* 1401–1405.

Moore, W. E. (1970). *Professions: Roles and rules.* New York, NY: Sage Foundation.

Moore-West, M., Testa, R.-M., & O'Donnell, J. F. (1998). A life in medicine: Stories from a Dartmouth medical school elective. *Academic Medicine, 73,* 153–159.

Morton, K., Lamberton, H. H., Testerman, J. K., Worthley, J. S., & Loo, L. K. (1996). Why does moral reasoning plateau during medical school? *Academic Medicine, 71,* 5–6.

Muller, S. C. (1984). Physicians for the twenty-first century: Report of the project panel on the general professional education of the physician and college preparation for medicine. *Journal of Medical Education, 59,* part 2.

Mullan, F. (1976). *White coat, clenched fist: The political education of an American physician.* New York, NY: Macmillan.

Nora, L. M., Daugherty, S. R., Mattis-Peterson, A., Stevenson, L., & Goodman, L. J. (1994). Improving cross-cultural skills of medical students through medical school–community partnerships. *Western Journal of Medicine, 161(2),* 144–147.

Novack, D., Epstein, R. M., & Paulsen, R. H. (1999). Toward creating physician-healers: Fostering medical students' self-awareness, personal growth, and well-being. *Academic Medicine, 74,* 516–520.

O'Neil, E. H., & Seifer, S. D. (1995). Health care reform and medical education: Forces toward generalism. *Academic Medicine, 70* (suppl. 1), 37–43.

Oransky, I., & Savitz, S. I. (1998, April 14). *USA Today,* p. 15A.

Oransky, I., & Savitz, S. I. (1998, April 14). Aloof medical students lack empathy for patients. *USA Today,* p. 15A.

Palepu, A., Friedman, R. H., Barnett, R. C., Carr, P. L., Ash, A. S., Szalacha, L., & Moskowitz, M. A. (1998). Junior faculty members' mentoring relationships and their professional development in U.S. medical schools. *Academic Medicine, 73* (3), 318–323.

Pappas, G., Hadden, W. C., Kozak, L. J., & Fisher, G. F. (1997). Potentially avoidable hospitalizations: Inequalities in rates between U.S. socioeconomic groups. *American Journal of Public Health, 87,* 811–816.

Pappas, G., Queen, S., Hadden, W., & Fisher, G. (1993). The increasing disparity in mortality between socioeconomic groups in the United States, 1960 and 1986. *New England Journal of Medicine, 329,* 103–109.

Pawlson, G. (1998). Rural and inner city outreach. *Meeting the needs of communities: How medical schools and teaching hospitals ensure access to clinical services.* Washington, DC: Association of American Medical Colleges.

Pellegrino, E. D., & Thomasma, D. C. (1981). *A philosophical basis of medical practice.* New York, NY: Oxford University Press.

Pellegrino, E. D., & Thomasma, D. C. (1993). *The virtues in medical practice.* New York, NY: Oxford University Press.

Pellegrino, E. D., Veatch, R. M., & Langan, J. P. (Eds). (1991). *Ethics, trust, and the professions.* Washington, DC: Georgetown University Press.

Petersdorf, R. G. (1992). Are we educating a medical professional who cares? *American Journal of Diseases of Children, 146,* 1338–1341.

Pew Health Professions Commission. (1994). *Primary care workforce 2000: Strategies for federal health policy reform.* San Francisco, CA: Pew Health Professions Commission.

Poehlman, G. S. (1999). Faculty workload assessment: A case study. *Family Medicine, 31,* 473–476.

Raelin, J. A. (1986). *The clash of cultures: Managers and professionals.* Boston, MA: Harvard Business School Press.

Rainey, C. (1997). Observations on the human cost of residency training. *Journal of the American Medical Association, 277,* 866.

Rappleye, W. C. (1932). *Medical education: Final report of the commission on medical education.* New York, NY: Association of American Medical Colleges.

Reilly, P. (1987). *To do no harm: A journey through medical school.* Dover, MA: Auburn House.

Reiser, S. J. (1994). The ethical life of health care organizations. *Hastings Center Report, 24(6),* 28–35.

Relman, A. (1998). Education to defend professional values in the new corporate age. *Academic Medicine, 73,* 1229–1233.

Rest, J. R. (1982). A psychologist looks at the teaching of ethics. *Hastings Center Report, 12(1),* 29–36.

Reuler, J. B., & Nardone, D. A. (1994). Role modeling in medical education. *Western Journal of Medicine, 160(4),* 335–337.

Reynolds, R., & Stone, J. (Eds.). (1995). *On doctoring.* New York, NY: Simon & Schuster.

Richards, R. W. (1990). Renewing medical education's social contract. *Israel Journal of Medical Science, 26,* 97–101.

Ring, J. J. (1991). The right road for medicine: Professionalism and the new American Medical Association. *Journal of the American Medical Association, 266,* 1694.

Rothman, D. J. (1991). *Strangers at the bedside.* New York, NY: Basic Books.

Rothstein, W. G. (1972). *American physicians in the nineteenth century: From sects to science.* Baltimore, MD: Johns Hopkins University Press.

Schein, E. H. (1992). *Organizational culture and leadership.* San Francisco, CA: Jossey-Bass.

Schiedermayer, D., & McCarthy, D. J. (1995). Altruism, professions, decorum, and greed: Perspectives on physician compensation. *Perspectives on Biology and Medicine, 38*, 238–253.

Schmidt, H. G., Neufeld, V. R., Nooman, Z. M., & Ogunbode, T. (1991). Network of community-oriented educational institutions for the health sciences. *Academic Medicine, 66*, 259–263.

Schroeder, S. A. (1992). The troubled profession: Is medicine's glass half full or half empty? *Annals of Internal Medicine, 116*, 583–592.

Schroeder, S. A, Jones, Z. S., & Showstack, J. A. (1989). Academic medicine as a public trust. *Academic Medicine, 262*, 803–812.

Scutchfield, F. D. (1998). The role of the medical profession in physician discipline. *Journal of the American Medical Association, 279*, 1915–1916.

Seifer, S. D. (1998). Service learning: Community-campus partnerships for health professions education. *Academic Medicine, 73*, 273–277.

Seifer, S. D., Mutha, S., & Connors, K. (1996). Service learning in health professions education: Barriers, facilitators and strategies for success. *Expanding Boundaries: Service and Learning, 1*, 36.

Sekas, G., & Hutson, W. R. (1995). Misrepresentation of academic accomplishments by applicants for gastroenterology fellowships. *Annals of Internal Medicine, 123*, 38–41.

Self, D. J., Olivarez, M., & Baldwin, D. C. J. (1998). Clarifying the relationship of medical education and moral development. *Academic Medicine, 73*, 517–520.

Self, D. J., Schrader, D. E., Baldwin, D. W. C., & Wolinsky, F. D. (1993). The moral development of medical students. A pilot study of the possible influences of medical education. *Medical Education, 27*, 26–34.

Self, D. J., Wolinsky, F. D., Baldwin, D. W. C., & Nease, D. E. (1989). The effect of teaching medical ethics on medical students' "moral reasoning." *Academic Medicine, 64*, 755–759.

Sheehan, K. H., Sheehan, D. V., White, K., Leibovitz, A., & Baldwin, D. C. (1990). A pilot study of medical student "abuse": Student perceptions of mistreatment and misconduct in medical school. *Journal of the American Medical Association, 263*, 533–537.

Shem, S. (1978). *The house of God*. New York, NY: Dell.

Shine, K. I. (1996). Educating physicians for the real world. In E. Ginzberg (Ed.), *Urban medical centers: Balancing academic and patient care functions* (pp. 5–11). Boulder, CO: Westview Press.

Shreves, J. G., & Moss, A. H. (1996). Residents' ethical disagreements with attending physicians: An unrecognized problem. *Academic Medicine, 71*, 1103–1105.

Shryock, R. H. (1967). *Medical licensing in America, 1650–1965*. Baltimore, MD: Johns Hopkins University Press.

Shugars, D. A., O'Neil, E. H., & Bade, J. D. (Eds.). (1991). *Healthy America: Practitioners for 2005, an agenda for action for U.S. health professional schools*. Durham, NC: Pew Health Professions Commission.

Sigerist, H. E. (1935). The history of medical licensure. *Journal of the American Medical Association, 104*, 1057–1060.

Skeff, K. M. & Mutha, S. (1998). Role models — guiding the future of medicine. *New England Journal of Medicine, 339*, 2015–2017.

Souba, W. W. (1996). Professionalism, responsibility and service in academic medicine. *Surgery, 119*, 1–8.

Southon, G., & Braithwaite, J. (1998). The end of professionalism. *Social Science and Medicine 46*, 23–28.

Stamos, D. (1996). Medical education in the u.s.: A student perspective. *Advisor, 16*, 32–39.

Starr, P. E. (1982). *The social transformation of American medicine: The rise of a sovereign profession and the making of a vast industry*. New York, NY: Basic Books.

Steele, D. J., & Susman, J. L. (1998). Integrated clinical experience: University of Nebraska Medical Center. *Academic Medicine, 73*, 41–47.

Stern, D. T. (1996). Hanging out: Teaching values in medical education. Unpublished doctoral dissertation, Stanford University.

Stern, D. T. (1996). Values on call: Methods for assessing the teaching of professionalism. *Academic Medicine, 71*, S37–S39.

Stevens, R. (1971). *American medicine and the public interest*. New Haven, CT: Yale University Press.

Stone, D. (1997). The doctor as businessman: The changing politics of a cultural icon. *Journal of Health Politics, Policy and Law, 22*, 533–556.

Sulmasy, D. P. (1999). Is medicine a spiritual practice? *Academic Medicine, 74*, 1002–1005.

Swick, H. M. (1998). Academic medicine must deal with the clash of business and professional values. *Academic Medicine, 73*, 751–755.

Swick, H. M., & Simpson, D. E. (1998). Letters to the editor: Another professional-skills course worth noting. *Academic Medicine, 73*, 725.

Tanouye. E. (1998a, November 16). Steep markups on generics top branded drugs. *Wall Street Journal*, pp. B1, B3.

Tanouye, E. (1998b, December 31). u.s. has developed an expensive habit; Now, how to pay for it? Scores of pricey new pills improve quality of life, but bust health budgets: Toenail-fungus cure: $500. *Wall Street Journal*, pp. A1, A10.

Taylor, C. (1991). *The ethics of authenticity*. Cambridge, MA: Harvard University Press.

Thompson, D. A., Petersen, M. C., & Boker, J. R. (1999). A longitudinal community clinical program for first-year medical students. *Academic Medicine, 74*, 600–601.

Todd, J. S. (1991). Professionalism at its worst. *Journal of the American Medical Association, 266*, 3338.

Toews, J. A., Lockyer, J. M., Dobson, D. J. G., Simpson, E., Brownell, A. K. W., Brenneis, F., MacPherson, K. M., & Cohen, G. S. (1997). Analysis of stress levels among medical students, residents, and graduate students at four Canadian schools of medicine. *Academic Medicine, 72*, 997–1002.

Towle, A. (Ed.). (1992). *Community-based teaching: Sharing ideas 1*. London, UK: King's Fund Centre.

United States Department of Health and Human Services (1997). *Preventing infant mortality* [On-line]. Available: http://www.healthystart.net/factsheet.html.

USA Snapshots. (1999, January 27). Doubts about managed care. *USA Today*, p. A1.

Wallace, A. G. (1997). Educating tomorrow's doctors: The thing that really matters is that we care. *Academic Medicine, 72*, 253–258.

Wallerstein, N. (1992). Powerlessness, empowerment, and health: Implications for health promotion programs. *American Journal of Health Promotion, 6*, 197–205.

Walton, H. J. (Ed.). (1993). Proceedings of the World Summit on Medical Education. *Medical Education, 28* (suppl. 1), 140–149.

Wasylenki, D., Byrne, N., & McRobb, B. (1997a). A pivotal agency model for community-based undergraduate medical education. *Education for Health, 10*, 311–318.

Wasylenki, D., Byrne, N., & McRobb, B. (1997b). The social contract challenge in medical education. *Medical Education, 31*, 250–258.

Wasylenki, D., Cohen, C., & McRobb, B. (1997c). Creating community agency placements for undergraduate medical education: A program description. *Canadian Medical Association Journal, 156(3)*, 379–383.

Watson, R., & Romrell, L. (1999). Mission-based budgeting: Removing a graveyard. *Academic Medicine, 74*, 627–640.

Ways, P. O. (1997). Interview by H. Brody & M. Halvorson. East Lansing, MI: Michican State University.

Ways, P. O., Loftus, G., & Jones, J. M. (1973). Problem teaching in medical education. *Journal of Medical Education, 48(6)*, 565–571.

Wear, D. (1997). Professional development of medical students: Problems and promises. *Academic Medicine, 72*, 1056–1062.

Weber, J. (1998, November 13). The doctor vs. the drugmaker: A dispute over a drug's efficacy turns a partnership into war. *Business Week*, 87–88.

Weiss, C., & Clamp, C. (1992). Women's cooperatives: Part of the answer to poverty? In L. Krimerman & F. Lindenfeld (Eds.), *When workers decide* (pp. 225–228). Philadelphia, PA: New Society Publishers.

White, K. L., & Connelly, J. E. (Eds.). (1992). *The medical school's mission and the population's health*. New York, NY: Springer Verlag.

Wilkes, M., Usatine, R., Slavin, S., & Hoffman, J. R. (1998). Doctoring: University of California, Los Angeles. *Academic Medicine, 73*, 32–40.

Wolgast, E. (1992). *Ethics of an artificial person: Lost responsibility in professions and organizations*. Stanford, CA: Stanford University Press.

Wong, J. (1999). Medical student's lament. *Body Electric, 15*, 6. (Literary arts magazine from University of Illinois College of Medicine-Chicago).

Wood, D. L. (1998). Educating physicians for the twenty-first century. *Academic Medicine, 73*, 1280–1281.

Wright, S. M., Kern, D. E., Kolodner, K., Howard, D. M., & Brancati, F. L. (1998). Attributes of excellent attending-physician role models. *New England Journal of Medicine, 339*, 1986–1993.

The Yale oath. (1994). *Yale Medicine*, Summer, 43.

Yankelovich, D. (1981, April). New rules in American life: Searching for self-fulfillment in a world turned upside down. *Psychology Today*, 35–91.

Zoloth-Dorfman, L., & Rubin, S. (1995). The patient as commodity: Managed care and the question of ethics. *Journal of Clinical Ethics, 6*, 339–356.

CONTRIBUTORS

Judith Andre, PH.D., is a professor of philosophy at Michigan State University in the Center for Ethics and Humanities in the Life Sciences and in the Philosophy Department. Her current research looks at the moral dimensions of professional life within the medical humanities, including what projects should be chosen, methods used, and communities formed.

Janet Bickel, M.A. has worked on issues of medical student and faculty professional development at the Association of American Medical Colleges for the last twenty-three years. In addition to publishing on a broad spectrum of areas in academic medicine, she has spoken at more than sixty-five schools and created a series of leadership-development seminars for women faculty. She began her involvement with medical education at Brown University, where from 1972 to 1976 she served as admissions, financial aid, and student affairs officer for the new medical school. She is the author of *Women in Medicine: Getting In, Surviving, and Advancing*.

The Bridging the Gaps Network is made up of faculty and staff from seven academic health centers in Pennsylvania, including Lake Erie College of Osteopathic Medicine, MCP Hahnemann University, Philadelphia College of Osteopathic Medicine, Temple University, Thomas Jefferson University, University of Pennsylvania, and the University of Pittsburgh. This group has worked together to develop and implement the Bridging the Gaps Program at each of their institutions. Their chapter is the result of the combined work of the network. The three lead authors are Lucy Wolf Tuton, PH.D., who serves as executive director of the overall program and has been involved in the development and implementation of the program since its inception in 1991; Claudia Siegel, M.A., M.P.A., who served as a Bridging the Gaps coordinator at two of the component programs before becoming consultant to Bridging the Gaps, responsible primarily for program evaluation; and Timothy Campbell, B.A., B.S.N., who is the overall program coordinator, providing the central administrative function to the state-wide initiative.

Howard Brody, M.D., PH.D., teaches in the Center for Ethics and Humanities in the Life Sciences and the Department of Family Practice at Michigan State University, East Lansing. The main focus of his work has been medical ethics. He is the author of *The Healer's Power* (1992) and *Stories of Sickness* (1987).

P. Niall Byrne, PH.D., is emeritus professor in the Centre for Research in Education, University of Toronto, Faculty of Medicine. His academic interests include international research and development, and the health effects of poverty on children. He is the director of a second-year undergraduate medical course, Health, Illness, and the Community.

Jordan J. Cohen, M.D., president and CEO of the Association of American Medical Colleges, is the chief advocate for academic medicine in the United States. His charge is to advance the positions of medical schools and teaching hospitals with the White

House, federal agencies, and the Congress. He has served as dean at the State University of New York at Stony Brook and has had faculty appointments at the University of Chicago, Tufts, Brown, and Harvard Medical Schools.

Jack Coulehan, M.D., M.P.H., is professor of preventive medicine at the State University of New York at Stony Brook, where he also directs the Institute for Medicine in Contemporary Society and chairs the university hospital ethics committee. He has written two volumes of poetry, *The Knitted Glove* (1991) and *First Photographs of Heaven* (1994), along with *The Medical Interview: Mastering Skills for Clinical Practice* (1997), a widely used text on the clinician-patient relationship, and *Blood and Bone* (coedited with Angela Belli, 1998), an anthology of poetry by physicians.

Edward J. Eckenfels is emeritus professor at Rush Medical College in Chicago where he served as the associate chairperson of the Department of Preventive Medicine and head of the Section of Community Health and Social Medicine. In addition, he was the first director of the Rush Community Service Initiatives Program. Over the past thirty years he has applied his conceptual knowledge and methodological skills to the study and teaching of social medicine and community health, the health care system, and medical education.

Jake Foglio, D.MIN., is assistant professor in the Department of Family Practice, a Catholic priest who has been a campus minister at Michigan State University for thirty years, and a teacher of spirituality for the last fourteen years in the College of Human Medicine at MSU. He developed a spirituality curriculum that has been incorporated into a required humanities block for second-year medical students at Michigan State University, and a required course on spirituality for interns in the Saint Lawrence Family Practice Residency Program in Lansing, Michigan.

Sue E. Fosson, M.A., is currently assistant dean for student affairs at the University of Kentucky College of Medicine. She has been at the University of Kentucky since 1974, beginning as an educational consultant in curriculum and evaluation. Since 1984 she has been working directly with medical students and assisting in their professional development.

Tana Grady-Weliky, M.D., is assistant professor of psychiatry and associate dean of undergraduate medical education at the University of Rochester School of Medicine and Dentistry. Her research interests include depression in women and minority populations, women's mental health issues, and obsessive-compulsive disorder. In addition to her work in undergraduate medical education, she is actively involved in psychiatric education for mental health professions and the community.

Frederic W. Hafferty, PH.D., is professor of behavioral sciences at the University of Minnesota-Duluth, School of Medicine. His current research focuses on the hidden curriculum in medical education, the role of trust in the ideology of professionalism, the social dimensions of medical effectiveness research, disability studies, and rural health issues.

Edward M. Hundert, M.D., is professor of psychiatry and medical humanities and senior associate dean for medical education at the University of Rochester School of Medicine and Dentistry, where he is leading a major curriculum reform called the Double Helix Curriculum, designed in part to ameliorate the potential for conflicting messages between the formal and the informal curricula.

Mary Anne Johnston, PH.D., is assistant professor of medicine in the Office of Education at the University of Colorado Health Sciences Center, where she provides educational programs and services to faculty in all health professions schools.

Cynthia N. Kettyle, M.D., is director of medical student education in the Department of Psychiatry at Harvard Medical School. In addition to her teaching and administrative responsibilities, she maintains a clinical practice of adult psychiatry and psychoanalysis.

Richard Martinez, M.D., is on the faculty of the Program in Health Care Ethics, Humanities, and Law at the University of Colorado Health Sciences Center. He directs the curriculum in ethics and humanities for the medical school, and has written in various journals and books on professional ethics and medical education.

Barbara McRobb is manager of community programs, University of Toronto, Faculty of Medicine. Her interests include community-based education, curriculum development, interprofessional education, and professionalism in medicine.

William D. Melton, M.D., currently splits time between La Clinca de la Raza and the Native American Health Center in Oakland, California, and Southern Humboldt Community Hospital in Garberville, California. He received a medical degree from the University of California, San Francisco, and completed a residency in family and community medicine at the University of New Mexico in Albuquerque.

Rick Miller received his medical degree from the University of California, San Francisco, and an M.P.H. from University of California-Berkeley in qualitative methods in public health. His interests before, during, and after medical training have been in working with local communities on health-related projects. He currently works as a family

practitioner with the Indian Health Service in Zuni, New Mexico, and is an assistant clinical professor at the University of New Mexico School of Medicine.

Lois Margaret Nora, M.D., J.D., is associate dean for academic affairs and administration at the University of Kentucky College of Medicine, where she is responsible for the undergraduate educational mission and faculty affairs. She graduated from Rush Medical College and the University of Chicago Law School.

Stanley Joel Reiser, M.D., PH.D., is the Griff T. Ross Professor of Humanities and Technology in Health Care at the University of Texas–Houston Health Science Center. He received his undergraduate education at Columbia University, his medical degree from the State University of New York-Downstate Medical Center, and his master's and doctoral degrees from Harvard University. His scholarship and teaching focus on ethics, technology assessment, history, and health policy.

Norma Wagoner, PH.D., is dean of students at the University of Chicago Pritzker School of Medicine and professor of organismal biology and anatomy. Her interests include the residency selection process, minority admissions, financial aid, and issues of humanism and professionalism.

Howard Waitzkin, M.D., M.P.H., is professor and director, Division of Community Medicine, Department of Family and Community Medicine, University of New Mexico. Author of *The Politics of Medical Encounters: How Patients and Doctors Deal with Social Problems*, he is interested in health policy, community medicine, and patient-doctor communication.

Donald Wasylenki, M.D., is professor of psychiatry and health administration in the Faculty of Medicine at the University of Toronto. He also holds the Foundation Baxter and Alma Ricard Chair in Inner City Health at Saint Michael's Hospital. From 1993 until 1998 he was founder and director of the Health, Illness and the Community course in the undergraduate medical curriculum at the University of Toronto.

Delese Wear is on the faculty at the Northeastern Ohio Universities College of Medicine in both the Human Values in Medicine and the Women and Medicine programs. She has written extensively on philosophical and curricular issues in professional development in medical education, and is the author or editor of three other books, including *Literary Anatomies: Women's Bodies and Health in Literature*; *Women in Medical Education: An Anthology of Experience*; and *Privilege in the Medical Academy: A Feminist Examines Gender, Race, and Power*. Her interests include medical humanities and women's health. She is the current editor of the *Journal of Medical Humanities*.

Peter Williams, J.D., M.P.H., is head of the Division of Medicine and Society, Department of Preventive Medicine, and vice dean for academic affairs at the State University of New York at Stony Brook. His teaching and scholarly interests include medical ethics and jurisprudence.

Sheila Woods, M.D., is a faculty member, director of the Adolescent Clinic at the Family Care Center, and medical director of the Professionalism Project in the Office of Academic Affairs for the University of Kentucky College of Medicine. This project seeks to inculcate professionalism and humanism in medical students, residents, and faculty through various curricular changes, extracurricular projects, and assessment strategies.

INDEX

humanities, 15, 27, 32, 49, 56, 57, 62, 63, 66, 67, 69, 84, 85, 93

Hunt, Andrew, 27, 82

institutional critics, 36, 37, 39, 42, 44, 47, 48

JAMA (Journal of the American Medical Association), 15, 22, 23

Kaplan, Stanley, x, 32–33
Kellogg Foundation, 134
Kierkegaard, Søren, 44
Klass, Perri, 31, 50
Kohlberg, Lawrence, 86
Koop, C. Everett, 23

LCME (Liaison Committee on Medical Education), 16, 27, 84, 129, 132; *Medical Education Database*, 17, 27; "The Structure and Function of the Medical School," 16, 27
Lundberg, George, 23, 34n

managed care, 11, 14, 17, 19, 29, 36, 46, 59, 65, 66, 68, 75, 96, 120, 132
MCAT, 32, 66, 118
Medicaid, 14, 54
medical educators, 3, 4, 5, 16, 26, 29, 30, 48, 56, 76, 77–78, 105–119, 123, 124, 125, 129, 132, 144, 147, 152, 185–191
medical school/clinical environment, 6, 24, 28, 30, 31, 37, 54, 55, 62, 99, 100, 101, 120, 122, 126, 129, 184, 186
medical students, 3, 4, 5; abuse of, 34n, 56, 129
Medicare, 14, 54
mentor/mentee, 58, 105–119, 120, 129–130, 167, 178, 186, 190
Merton, Thomas, 81, 91
mission statements, 10, 11, 29, 30, 122, 167
mistakes in medicine, 87–88, 186
moral behavior, 38
moral climate, 48
moral development and growth, 27, 86, 90, 94
moral reasoning, 80, 86, 89, 91
morality, 27, 39

multiculturalism, 97–98, 99–101, 121, 128, 141–142, 166, 167, 175, 188

needs assessment, 76, 136
NEJM (New England Journal of Medicine), 14

oath, 103
orientation, 125, 126

patient-physician covenant, 96
pedagogy, 24
Pellegrino, Edmund, 54
Percival, Thomas, 57
personal growth, 16
Pew Health Professions Commission, 110, 151, 167
physician-patient relationship, 15, 20, 21, 24, 51, 56, 63, 84, 116, 178, 185, 190
population-based medicine, 15
power, 29, 56, 69
Princeton Review, x, 32
professional identity, 35, 37, 45, 56
professional role, 35–48
professionalism/professional development, 3, 13, 14, 15, 16, 17, 19, 20, 21, 22, 23, 28, 29, 30, 32, 33, 35, 44, 48, 54, 55, 56, 57, 68, 73, 74, 75, 78, 79, 80, 85, 86, 95, 96, 98, 101, 103, 104, 105–119, 120, 121, 124, 126, 128, 129, 132, 174, 180, 182, 184–191; components of, 18, 23, 27, 30, 50, 51, 52, 54, 56, 58, 59, 60, 65, 66, 68, 76, 80, 93, 95, 120, 132, 167, 173; evaluation/measurement of, 78, 79, 129, 132, 185–186; history of, 14–16, 121; nonreflective, 58, 59, 60, 61, 62, 64, 65, 69
proletarianization, 21

reflection, 30, 31, 80, 94, 104, 126, 131, 146, 173, 189, 190
Relman, Arnold, 13, 18, 19, 23
residency, 42, 79, 93, 131, 134–149
Robert Wood Johnson Foundation, 23, 125, 151, 167
role models, 103, 106, 129–130, 185

sexual orientation, 101–103
Shem, Samuel, 31
social activism, 51, 69, 129, 130, 134–149, 166, 184
socialization, 11, 14, 31, 55, 57, 59, 60, 168
socioeconomic status, 134, 135, 136–137, 141, 147–149, 151, 165, 174, 177–178, 187
sociology, 19–21, 22
spirituality, 81, 85, 89–94, 191

tacit learning, 52, 56, 57, 60, 63
Taylor, Charles, 43, 44

Thomasma, David, 54
trust, 22, 138, 187

unprofessional behavior, 24–25, 26, 39, 77, 101–103, 122, 123, 132, 185
USMLE, 32, 34 n, 126, 127

virtues, 22, 51, 53–55, 59, 60, 64, 91, 93
volunteerism, 53, 167, 171–173

Ways, Peter, 83
white coat ceremony, 80, 125